Register Now for Online Access to Your Book!

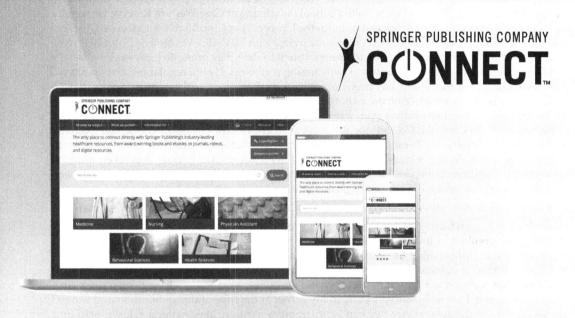

Joseph Perazzo, PhD, RN, ACRN, graduated from Xavier University with a bachelor of science in psychology and completed his nursing degree from Xavier's Master of Nursing Direct Entry as Second Degree (MIDAS) program. He completed a PhD in nursing from the University of Cincinnati College of Nursing and completed an National Institutes of Health T32 postdoctoral fellowship in symptom science from Frances Payne Bolton School of Nursing at Case Western Reserve University. He is currently an assistant professor of nursing at the University of Cincinnati with a focused research program dedicated to health promotion in people living with HIV. Dr. Perazzo has published more than 25 articles in peer-reviewed scientific publications to date, has presented his work nationally and internationally, and has contributed to two nursing textbooks. He is a regular reviewer for seven peer reviewed publications and has been recognized by Publons for his contribution as a peer-reviewer. He is also a member of the editorial board of the *Journal of the Association of Nurses in AIDS Care (JANAC)* and an abstract reviewer for the American Nurses Foundation, the Association of Nurses in AIDS Care, the Council for the Advancement of Nursing Science, and the Midwest Nurse Research Society. Dr. Perazzo has mentored undergraduate and graduate nursing students, including master's, doctor of nursing practice, and PhD students. Dr. Perazzo has taken multiple graduate-level writing courses and has attended multiple grant and manuscript writing workshops from writing experts, and has a long-term goal of editing for scientific publications.

And now the rest of the story . . .

I was absolutely convinced that I was never going to be able to publish a paper. My first attempt at publication resulted in four sequential rejections (which included rejections of revised previous rejections). I was disheartened because I liked writing, but this feedback made me feel like I was anything but good at it. I have had some wonderful mentors, and all of them told me (and continue to tell me) that rejection is a part of the process and that I just need to keep trying, keep practicing, and keep learning. I am still relatively early in my career at the time of this publication and wanted to pass on some of the great advice I've had in my training. Writing, like anything, takes a lot of time (and can be just plain tedious), but it can open up a lot of doors for you. Many times, there is nothing I would rather do *less* than sit at my computer and write, but in the end I am always glad that I did. I hope you enjoy this book and I wish you the very best!

—*Joe Perazzo*

Robert Topp, PhD, RN, graduated from the University of Toledo with a bachelor of science in nursing, from the University of Cincinnati with an MSN, from The Ohio State University with a PhD in health education and exercise physiology, and completed a 2-year postdoctoral fellowship in geriatric medicine at the University of Pennsylvania. Over his 28 years in academic nursing, he has been the principal investigator or coinvestigator on over $3 million of extramurally supported research projects, which has resulted in over 140 publications in peer-reviewed journals and over 300 presentations at professional scientific meetings. His expertise in the areas of research methodology and statistics is sought by numerous professional organizations and journals to review proposals for funding, manuscripts for publication, and abstracts for presentation. Finally, Dr. Topp has a consistent history of mentoring students and junior faculty in obtaining intra- and extramural awards and facilitating completion of their projects through to publication and presentation.

And now the rest of the story . . .

Early in my career, after reading a bio like the one you just read about me, I would become discouraged and depressed. I wondered how I was ever going to write so many articles when I was struggling to write just one. I would wonder what personal, physical, and/or mental sacrifices I would need to make in academic nursing, or whether productive authors are just lucky to be "born writers." After 28 years I realize that "luck" has nothing to do with being a productive author. The "secret sauce" to being a productive author is simply frequently sitting down, writing, revising, and incorporating critique. Although I have authored a number of articles, I have *never* had a manuscript accepted for publication without comments from reviewers and editors for changes that needed to be made before accepting it for publication. Further, a majority of my publications are the result of submitting a manuscript multiple times to multiple journals, which sometimes took years. Finally, I leave you with this quote:

"Luck has a lot to do with success and I've noticed that lucky people work hard and persevere."

—*Bob Topp*

PAIN-FREE WRITING FOR NURSES
A Step-by-Step Approach

Joseph Perazzo, PhD, RN, ACRN

Robert Topp, PhD, RN

SPRINGER PUBLISHING COMPANY

Springer Publishing Company, LLC
11 West 42nd Street
New York, NY 10036
www.springerpub.com
http://connect.springerpub.com

Acquisitions Editor: Joseph Morita
Compositor: S4Carlisle Publishing Services

ISBN: 978-0-8261-3987-0
e-book ISBN: 978-0-8261-3991-7
Faculty Guide ISBN: 978-0-8261-3973-3
DOI: 10.1891/9780826139917

Instructor's Materials: Qualified instructors may request supplements by emailing textbook @springerpub.com

19 20 21 22 / 5 4 3 2 1

The author and the publisher of this Work have made every effort to use sources believed to be reliable to provide information that is accurate and compatible with the standards generally accepted at the time of publication. The author and publisher shall not be liable for any special, consequential, or exemplary damages resulting, in whole or in part, from the readers' use of, or reliance on, the information contained in this book. The publisher has no responsibility for the persistence or accuracy of URLs for external or third-party Internet websites referred to in this publication and does not guarantee that any content on such websites is, or will remain, accurate or appropriate.

CIP data is on file at the Library of Congress.

Contact us to receive discount rates on bulk purchases.
We can also customize our books to meet your needs.
For more information please contact: sales@springerpub.com

Joseph Perazzo: https://orcid.org/0000-0002-9893-5247
Robert Topp: https://orcid.org/0000-0001-6667-5789

Publisher's Note: **New and used products purchased from third-party sellers are not guaranteed for quality, authenticity, or access to any included digital components.**

Printed in the United States of America.

To Jeff West: for always being my champion, my cheerleader, and my dearest friend.
—Joe Perazzo

To my Schmoochie (sweet wife Jamie), who completes me
—Bob Topp

CONTENTS

CONTRIBUTORS

Jennifer Avery, PhD, RN, GNP-BC   Assistant Professor of Nursing, Eastern Michigan University, Livonia, Michigan

Amanda Y. Makula, MA, BA   Digital Initiatives Librarian, University of San Diego, San Diego, California

Joseph Perazzo, PhD, RN, ACRN   Assistant Professor of Nursing, University of Cincinnati College of Nursing, Cincinnati, Ohio

Carol J. Scimone, BA   Executive Assistant, Office of Development, University of San Diego Hahn School of Nursing and Health Science, San Diego, California

Robert Topp, PhD, RN   Associate Dean for Research and Scholarship, College of Nursing, University of Toledo, Toledo, Ohio

David E. Vance, PhD, MGS   Interim Associate Dean for Research and Scholarship, Office of Research and Scholarship, School of Nursing, The University of Alabama at Birmingham, Birmingham, Alabama

FOREWORD

A major challenge for nurses, including faculty, clinicians, and students, has been, and continues to be, to engage in more scholarly writing. This book defines scholarly writing as writing that involves the transfer of new knowledge. The types of scholarly writing explored in the book are not limited to publications in research and practice journals, but also proposals, abstracts, letters, and articles in the popular press (including newspapers, magazines, blogs), and more. Knowledge moves through the discipline of nursing in many ways. The results of rigorous research that document effective and efficient strategies to improve patient outcomes are only widely available when the findings are published. The outcomes of evidence-based practice projects, quality improvement projects, or other scholarly projects are commonly reported only within the local organization where the project is conducted. Widely accessible publication of information about best practices is vital for those practices to be extensively distributed to improve the care for a larger number of patients. Publication is much more than a nice hobby when time is available; it is essential to improve patient outcomes. If you have knowledge that is not widely known, it is your professional responsibility to publish that knowledge. The value of this book is that it explains how to disseminate new knowledge to improve patient care.

I have been the editor-in-chief of one of the premier nursing research journals, *Western Journal of Nursing Research*, for many years. We receive over 400 manuscript submissions each year. Because journal space is limited, many manuscripts are rejected. Sometimes manuscripts that might be reporting valuable new knowledge are denied publication because the authors did not write clearly about their projects. Authors who have difficulty synthesizing previous knowledge, describing how their project was conducted and analyzed, interpreting findings in the context of practice and research, or describing how findings could be implemented in practice often receive journal rejection decisions. The peer review process allows for some clarification in revised manuscripts when the author submitted an excellent first submission. The journal review process typically does not accommodate authors of poorly crafted manuscripts. This book is an excellent resource for authors who want to publish their scholarly products. The book is especially insightful with strategies to avoid common pitfalls in the authorship trajectory.

I have known and worked with Dr. Topp for many years. We have conducted workshops related to scholarly writing. Dr. Topp has served on our journal editorial board for over a decade. He has extensive experience working with doctoral students and junior faculty as they hone their writing skills. He brings deep and broad expertise to this book. Dr. Perazzo is a rising star who has recent immediate experience developing his publication record during and after his postdoctoral fellowship. He has participated in local and national writing workshops, is a regular peer reviewer for multiple scientific journals, and is a member of the editorial board for the *Journal of the Association of Nurses in AIDS Care*. This editorship combination is a unique and dynamic feature of this book.

Scholarly writing skills matter. The good news is that scholarly writing skills can be learned. No one is born a good writer. This book wisely starts with an in-depth examination of strategies to overcome typical barriers to starting the writing process by acknowledging authorship ambivalence. I appreciate the chapter discussing title and abstract preparation. Too often, authors hastily construct these at the end of their writing process not realizing that editors and peer reviewers use the title and abstract to frame their expectations about the paper. I especially appreciate an entire chapter devoted to outline development; many writing problems can be prevented with a good outline. The book also addresses the challenge of revising papers as well as co-authorship issues. One chapter addresses the potential advantages of open access to authors' work. I would urge authors to be careful in pursuing open access publication venues. The predatory publication industry is inventive and enormous. Publication in reputable journals enhances project credibility while publication in disreputable outlets diminishes credibility and can damage professional reputations. Discussing open access publication venues with experienced authors is wise. One of the strengths of this book is its addressing of the diverse aspects of writing for publication.

You will enjoy seeing your scholarly writing widely disseminated and incorporated into improving patient care. Publication of your scholarly writing is personally satisfying. You will savor the feeling from knowing your ideas are widely influencing patient care. That really is the bottom line—we nurses through scholarly inquiry aim to generate new knowledge that will improve patient care. Scholarly writing is the process by which new knowledge is communicated.

Vicki S. Conn, PhD, RN, FAAN
Editor, *Western Journal of Nursing Research*
Professor Emerita
University of Missouri

PREFACE

Dear ~~Reader~~ Future Author!

Welcome! We are confident that you are opening this book because, like us, you have a hard time containing your excitement for writing. We pity people who fail to experience the exhilaration that comes with seeing a document emerge from a blank white screen. Some of us have our raison d'être in writing. Sometimes your friends, colleagues, and loved ones may say things like, "Better you than me!" or "I am so glad that I will never *ever* have to write a paper again" when you tell them about the work you do. Just know that they are jealous that it is not them. Okay, that was fun, so much for the "rah rah" of the introduction—and now back to reality.

Before you go any further, we want you to know that we understand if the very thought of writing conjures negative feelings of anxiety, anger, guilt, or self-loathing. Maybe you made the decision a long time ago that you do not write well and that you would rather have a root canal while staring at the sun than write a paper. We, the authors, your friendly colleagues in the scholarly world, met at a scientific conference . . . in the hotel bar. We were lamenting the topic of scholarly writing and sharing the different methods we used to be productive authors. We discussed the similar struggles we experienced with writing. In addition to finding a lot of common ground, we shared approaches we used to be more effective and productive authors. We agreed that we learned many of these tips, tricks, and resources through trial and error or informal sharing with our colleagues. After another round of "inspiration," we decided the world needed a book designed for nurses who are pursuing a graduate degree or took a job in academia. Thus, our project to write this book came to life.

In this book, we provide you with information that will temper your anxiety or hatred of writing and allow you to experience writing as a satisfying approach to expanding knowledge and not a painful chore to avoid. We have drawn from the work of writing and productivity experts and have invited a diverse group of productive scholars to contribute chapters on a variety of topics.

Throughout the book you will receive personal stories, advice,* and direction on scholarly writing processes, and writing tips appear in boxes throughout each chapter. At the end of each chapter, we provide

---

*Free advice is worth every nickel you pay for it.

you with annotated writing examples that are yours to "adopt." These examples can help you write different types of scholarly documents. We will present information on barriers to writing and some solutions you can use to get past them (Chapter 1), walk through the process of writing a scholarly paper (Chapter 2), and discuss ways to prepare and set yourself up to write successfully (Chapters 3–5). We wanted this book to be more than simply a "how to write guide" for writing data-based journal articles, since academic careers often require us to author a variety of scholarly documents. So we also have chapters dedicated to writing for employment (Chapter 6), giving, receiving and responding to feedback on your writing (Chapter 7), writing as part of a team (Chapter 8), writing difficult documents (Chapter 9), and some creative ways you can disseminate your work to others (Chapter 10). Finally, we have provided a chapter from a self-proclaimed "grammar cop" to help you with common missteps and mistakes with the technical aspects of writing (Chapter 11).

You may have any number of reasons for picking up this book: You may be a graduate student or a faculty member; you may be struggling to write a manuscript or letters of recommendation. If you find yourself frustrated with writing, you can read this book and find out that you are not alone. Writing skills are not the result of divine providence. No one is born writing well. Proficient writing, like making 43.8% of your 3-point shots in basketball, is the result of practicing the skill.[†] We hope that you will find this book helpful, and pull it off the shelf (or up on the screen) when you are struggling to get that writing done! Writing is as painful as you choose to make it. We hope that this book will be a tool you can use to make the task of writing a bit easier for yourself, and maybe—just maybe—find that you can actually enjoy writing.

Sincerely,

Joseph Perazzo, PhD, RN, ACRN
Robert Topp, PhD, RN

ACKNOWLEDGMENTS

We would like to acknowledge the tireless contributions of *everyone* who read the countless drafts of this manuscript and provided suggestions for improving it. Many unnamed people can take credit for the content and quality of this book, which was truly a group effort. Thank you all.

[†] Seth Curry's lifetime 3-point average as a result of practicing 2,000 3-point shots a week.

CHAPTER 1

REASONS NOT TO WRITE AND GETTING PAST THEM

Joseph Perazzo

PERSONAL STORY

"You know what?" my colleague exclaimed. "Life is too short for this! I don't even care anymore! I don't like writing, I'm terrible at it, and I am not trying to become an author or a researcher! I am a good nurse! Someone will hire me!" My coworker was inconsolable about a big writing assignment in one of her BSN classes. A nurse for over 30 years, she was suddenly faced with either getting her BSN or finding a new job. She was an amazing nurse and teacher and any of us who worked with her in the ICU would entrust our family members' care to her.

I had never seen her under such a high level of stress. This writing assignment had really taken a toll on her mentally, physically, and spiritually, while she was running out of time to submit it. She turned it in, earned a passing grade, and the world kept on turning. During the 2 years she needed to complete her degree, I saw her move in and out of this level of stress every time she had a writing assignment due. In the end, she completed the program and earned her BSN. Sometime later, another nurse complimented her on her excellent teaching ability and asked if she would ever considered becoming a faculty member at a nursing school. Without so much as a pause, she said, "I think it would be very fulfilling, but I will never darken the door of a school again. Not with all that writing. Sorry." Looking back, I see now that scholarly writing stood in the way of her potentially doing something she would have found fulfilling.

Years later, I completed my graduate school program and research fellowship. I worked with amazing faculty members, learned from writing and productivity experts, and developed a set of skills that have helped me to become a productive writer. I learned something

1

that I want to pass on to you—writing does not need to be something you dread; you are in control of how stressful it is. Wait! Before you close the book, please allow me to explain.

INTRODUCTION

Today, I can say that I enjoy writing, but do not be fooled; I am a work in progress and likely always will be. I still procrastinate. I still become overwhelmed and anxious because of projects, grants, and deadlines. I then avoid the task, which always comes back to bite me later. I put all my energy into *thinking* about writing and none of it into *actually* writing. However, I can say that I now have tools to help me get through those moments. One of the best decisions I made was to take time to read books by writing experts, attend writing workshops and courses, and understand my own thoughts, feelings, attitudes, and habits that were damaging my productivity. Tips from writers, academicians, and productivity experts like Joyce Fitzpatrick, Jean Goodson, Paul Silvia, Stephen King, and Neil Fiore have given me countless tools to improve my writing. I learned that I was responsible for much of the stress I felt when faced with a writing project but making small (but significant) changes made a world of difference. Whatever your reason for reading this book, I (along with all the other authors involved in this book) would like to pass along some of this advice to you. In this chapter, I discuss five common barriers to productive writing and offer some solutions to these barriers that may help you along the way.

BARRIER #1: A BAD ATTITUDE

I am the last person to admonish anyone who does not like to write. Writing requires time, patience, concentration, and self-discipline; these are things some of us do not have in abundance. Writing assignments may fill you with anxiety and even anger. They can make you resent the person who assigned it or even yourself for committing to do it. Before the pen hits the paper or your fingers hit the keys, many people have some (or all) of the following thoughts:

- I *hate* writing
- I am not a writer
- I am a terrible writer
- This is such a waste of time
- This is going to be AWFUL

I promise you that if you approach writing as a burden, it will *always* be one. Writing is a way of expressing valuable thoughts and knowledge and nurses have a lot of these treasures to share. You also may have different reasons for writing. It may be a paper for a class, a capstone project, a dissertation, a manuscript you hope to have published, a presentation for a professional conference, a memo, a letter, or some other project. Writing may not be your favorite activity, but it does not have to increase your blood pressure when you do it.

Solution: Turn Over a New Leaf and Get Some Practice!

Very few people are born writers, just as very few people are born athletes. At some point along the way, you develop skills. Most of the time, these skills are fostered with patience, perseverance, and practice. A great way to get your start is to make a commitment <u>now</u> to view writing differently. Negative self-talk and stewing about the injustice of the expectation to write are roadblocks to completing your writing task. When you start to slip into that kind of thinking, just remember why you originally chose to do what you are doing. An interesting paradox that I have seen in fellow nurses who struggle with writing is they are often some of the most interesting people I have ever known. Nurses are exposed to events that most people will never see. They can tell some amazing stories. In this book you will learn some tools that will help demystify the writing process, but no amount of advice will be helpful if you get in your own way.

Another great piece of advice is to train yourself on writing. Keep a journal or a blog that you update regularly. This does not require a lot of research and is a great way to practice getting words on paper or on the screen. Initially, do not obsess over language, grammar, or context. Your goal is to start working those writing muscles. Carve out time each day to write and commit to that block of time as if it were an appointment.

BARRIER #2: COUNTERPRODUCTIVE WRITING BEHAVIORS

The writing behaviors I am referring to are the *when*, *where*, and *how* of your writing. If you find that you struggle with the task of writing, it is well worth a self-appraisal to determine if you might be getting in your own way. In my case, I was an expert at rationalizing the way I chose to write (e.g., all night on the date an assignment was due even though I had 5 weeks to work on it). I would say things like, "I have to be in the right frame of mind to write" or "I am really the type that likes to dive in and get it all done at once. I thrive under pressure." The way I chose to write was physically and mentally exhausting, and the quality of my work suffered. I would get papers back from professors with big red question marks, just like in grammar school. In my desperation to finish the paper, I skipped vital information or (if I am completely honest) slipped into complete delirium and wrote sentence fragments or nonsense. I may have survived some term papers with this behavior, but I had to change my thought pattern to succeed in graduate school or a career in academia.

There are probably many ways people could describe their writing habits, but they often fall into two major categories: binge writing and piecemeal writing.

Binge Writing

For some people, scheduling a large chunk of time to immerse themselves in a writing project is best. They are able to maintain a high level of focus and feel productive using this method. However, binge writing rarely means a paper or manuscript is ready to submit in one sitting. Some people truly do best when they can plan for long stretches of time to write, even if they have to do it multiple times.

Piecemeal Writing

People who prefer this writing method may not be as successful when trying to write for a long stretch of time. Rather, they write for shorter (and likely more numerous) blocks of sustained writing time. They are able to return to the same writing project many times and methodically piece it together rather than immersing themselves in the task all at once. You may dance back and forth depending on the writing task, or perhaps you have not done enough writing to develop a preference yet. There is no one way to write. Only you know if *your* way works for you or if it is hurting your productivity.

Solution: An Honest Self-Assessment and a Calendar

There is something liberating about looking a problem in the eye and tackling it. I advise you to ask yourself the following questions:

- When and where am I most productive with my writing?
- Do I write better in a few long stretches or in multiple shorter time blocks?
- What have I done in the past that I do *not* want to repeat in the future? (This may be the most important question.)

Once you have answered these questions, you can act, and all you need is a calendar and a commitment. In nearly every writing book I have read, the authors talk about the need for a commitment to your protected writing time. Whether it is writing in long stretches a few afternoons each week or a short block of time every day, the real key to success is for you to learn to treat that block of time as you would <u>any other important commitment</u>. It is very easy to put off writing. But you do not put off picking up your children from school, an important appointment with the doctor, or teaching a class. These tasks are on your calendar with a certain nonnegotiable quality about them.

> **WRITING TIP**
> Don't allow others to set your priorities for you. Remember, it will be *your* time that is spent making up for it!

Once you learn to commit to protecting these blocks of time for your writing, it will become habit. The easiest way to make this a reality is to get it on the calendar and make yourself unavailable to others during that time. Think of it like this: Writing just one completed paragraph a week could yield multiple papers or manuscripts in a year! If you are writing a class paper, start as soon as possible to give yourself plenty of time. If you want to publish your research, set up a plan and stick to it!

BARRIER #3: LACK OF PREPARATION

If you are like me, you might have a history of writing binges that lasted into the wee hours of the morning in a frantic effort to finish an assignment. A writing workshop I attended had an entire breakout session on the importance of the preparatory phase of writing. The facilitator pointedly described what writing is like when you fail to prepare, and it was a precise description of my experience.

One reason my writing was an exhausting marathon was because I was doing a lot more than just writing. In one sitting I would be doing background research online, switching windows frequently to find information needed to write my paper. I would also try to write the paper from beginning to end perfectly so there was no need to edit. This led to ridiculously long blocks of time perfecting one sentence or paragraph. The actual writing process, therefore, was incredibly difficult and would lead me to burnout and frustration. To top it all off, I learned that I was often creating more work for myself later. Renowned writer Anne Lamott (1995), in her book *Bird by Bird*, has a chapter called "Shitty First Drafts":

> "All good writers write them," Lamott says. "This is how they end up with good second drafts and terrific third drafts."

Many authors believe that writing really begins during the editing phase. Your first draft gets the information down on paper. Subsequent drafts perfect the style, grammar, and punctuation.

Solution: Work Smart and Give Yourself Some Credit!

In addition to the writing templates discussed in this book, you will be given templates for a variety of documents that will make the process much easier. In-depth advice on creating these documents will be covered in other chapters, but here are some key steps to remember in the preparatory phase of writing:

- Always start with an outline of what you want to accomplish. (See Chapter 4, Everything Begins and Ends With an Outline, on how to create an effective outline and optimize your use of it.)

- Do the research necessary for the paper (e.g., background research, data analyses) before you begin writing; add the key points and citations to your outline.

- Continually refine your outline as you research so you have a single document as a reference while you are writing your narrative.

- Commit to getting the words on the paper; you can edit later

- Sometimes you will struggle to find the right thing to say. Do not waste time believing you have hit a wall. You have not! You will dress this part up later. Think of writing like a sculpture: It is beautiful in the end but starts as a big hunk of nonsense.

While you may not feel productive during the preparatory phase of writing because you are not composing *the* narrative you will submit, give yourself the credit you are due! As pointed out by several writing experts, these preparatory steps are what give you the substance for your writing (Goodson, 2017; King, 2002; Silvia, 2007). Furthermore, your narrative will be more organized, come together more quickly, and *possibly* require fewer revisions.

BARRIER #4: "TIME IS JUST NOT ON MY SIDE"

> **WRITING TIP**
> Track the amount of time you think or worry about writing. Now track the time you spend writing. Surprising, isn't it? You're welcome.

There is no sense in pretending that writing is quick and easy! It often takes a substantial amount of time. Some writing assignments are like bad pennies that stick around despite our wishes for them to go away. I realized during my first job out of graduate school that if I ever wanted to sleep more than 2 hours per night, something needed to change. I always felt so short on time. I would be willing to bet that a perceived lack of time to write is one, if not the most commonly cited, reason people have difficulty writing. This is a good time to revisit the different types of writing behavior: binge writing and piecemeal writing. As I stated previously, if you are a successful, productive binge writer, my hat is off to you. However, it is often difficult to find long stretches of time to write. When these times do appear in our schedules it can be difficult to put writing ahead of more pleasurable activities.

When facing a large, sticky web of deadlines in every direction, people will often fall on their sword and describe themselves as procrastinators (as though procrastination is a cardinal trait). I am certainly guilty of this. Sometimes I go into a project with the very best of intentions only to be humbled by the need to apologize to my team members, ask for extensions, and make a host of new promises for getting the project done. Now for the cold hard truth: It is true that I have submitted projects late or failed to complete a task because of an overwhelming workload or a personal crisis. However, I have also submitted projects late because of Netflix binges, leisure reading, long naps, movies, and sometimes even long stretches of "doing nothing at all" time. It is amazing how clean my house and car become when I am avoiding a paper.

> **WRITING TIP**
> *"Insanity is doing the same thing over and over again and expecting a different result"*
>
> –Unknown

While I kick myself for being late, I have learned why I do it. First, leisure is necessary. It is helps us refuel and recharge. However, I learned a lot about procrastination reading Neil Fiore's (2007) book on productivity. Fiore takes a different perspective than most on procrastination. Typically, people beat themselves up and look at their procrastination as a character weakness. Fiore points out the reality is that procrastination should come as no surprise; that people procrastinate because it can feel rewarding. When we procrastinate, we get the temporary reward feeling of avoiding the unpleasantness of writing. After all, it can wait, right? There is an entire week before it is due! The problem, of course, is when you go through this process repeatedly, the avoided task becomes bigger and more menacing. Finally, you have no choice but to face it and by the time you finish you vow to never again procrastinate. Often, however, once that assignment or manuscript becomes a memory and a new one comes along, procrastination shows up to taunt us. As Sméagol from "Lord of the Rings" might say, "You have plenty of time, my love! Check out this new British crime series on Netflix." At the end of the day, you are human, and when faced with the choice of doing something pleasant or something unpleasant, the decision is often not a difficult one.

Solution: Stop Choosing Work or Life and Give Yourself Both!

The best piece of advice I have been given is to work hard but to remember there is more to life than how many articles you write. You have to live your life, have fun, and experience good things. A busy academic program or career that involves working your intellectual muscles can make you feel like there is never enough time. Even when you are not technically working you may continue to brainstorm. Furthermore, you may have a lot of serious commitments going on in your life that add obstacles and complications to time management. Whether you believe me or not, writing does not have to be one of those complications. Taking some of the suggestions you will find in this book will help you not only with the writing itself, but how to integrate the writing into your life. While only you know your priorities, here are some writing suggestions I have heard that help authors to manage their time and write more efficiently:

- Write a few paragraphs or for 30 minutes as the very first task of each day. That way if the day becomes hectic with classes, meetings, kids, appointments, and so on, you can meet those demands knowing you have already accomplished some writing. This may mean you will have to commit to getting up earlier than usual or combining your writing time with your morning coffee.

- Buy a small digital recorder and talk it out! This solution is perfect for those who get their best writing ideas when they are in the car, at night in bed, or at other "random" times. This helps to at least save the idea so when you sit down to write you do not end up staring at a blank page.

- Go to jail—by jail, I do not mean *actual* jail. However, you may prefer it to this suggestion (but remember you are turning over a new leaf). This idea comes from academics who would put themselves in "grant jail." We do this at my workplace and it is very effective. Placing a sign on your door, cubical, or desk that says "grant jail," "dissertation jail," or "manuscript jail," allows others to see that you are engaged in important writing work and cannot be interrupted.

- Insulate yourself. During your writing time make the following customary: no office or cell phone; no Internet or email; no Snapchat, Facebook, Instagram, or Twitter. It is just you, your research, and the computer.

- *Put it on an actual calendar (not just the one in your mind).* I am most emphatic about this last suggestion because it is, arguably, the most widely recommended by experts (Goodson, 2017; Silvia, 2007). In general, people do not put a lot of tasks on the calendar that they can easily push off to another time. In today's world of technology, people can block off time from their calendar that will not only notify them and send them reminders but it will let others know, "Sorry, no meeting time available!"

Regardless of your specific method, the take-home point of this section is to choose a way to integrate writing into your life that truly works for you. Of greater importance, once you find the way that works for you, you must protect that time as you would other commitments. In

> **WRITING TIP**
> I envy your multitasking abilities.
> You can "work so well under
> pressure" *and* be "so stressed out"
> all at the same time! Amazing!

addition to being easy to push off, it is often easy for others to try to poach writing time. This is often not intentional, but it is an easy task to resume later. As anyone who writes knows "later" may never arrive! Do not be afraid to discuss this commitment with friends, family, and colleagues who will support and respect your time. Give these methods a try and you may be surprised how much more quickly and easily your writing takes shape and comes to life than it has before.

BARRIER #5: FEAR

Fear is a major writing barrier for many people. Often, it comes down to the realization that reason we write is for others to read our work! Writing involves the sharing of information, ideas, and perspectives and opening them up for someone else to read. Whether you really care about an assignment or a paper, it is something you created. It is personal. You spent time on it. I had a professor during my freshman year in college give me a very harsh critique of a paper. He tore everything to shreds, from my sentence structure to the content of my ideas. I felt angry and even hurt by this feedback. You may have had similar experiences, and I do not blame you for not wanting to go through it again.

As you will read many times in this book, writing is a way of joining an ongoing conversation and feedback is a part of that process (see Chapter 7, Responding to Feedback). Even the most experienced scientists admit that when they press the "submit" button for a grant or a manuscript, they briefly fantasize about having the submission reviewed glowingly and processed without further revisions. Everyone wants one type of feedback on their work, the one that goes like this: "I could not find *anything* wrong with this! It is a true masterpiece that has changed my life for the better. Bravo!" Dare to dream, my friend. Whether it is a nursing graduate student or a famous novelist, everyone gets a bit antsy about how their work will be perceived.

Solution: Use This Book!

Fear not! There are many reasons my coauthor and I decided to write a book about writing for nurses. Above all, we reflected on the fact that there are opportunities abundant academically, clinically, and in the community, and more opportunities are being presented for nurses to return to school and pursue advanced degrees. We knew firsthand that writing was not a skill heavily emphasized in the clinical setting. Many nurses return to school and hit a roadblock when they are assigned a paper to write. Even those we work with in academia sometimes struggle with the expectations of scholarly writing. It is our hope that when you are frustrated, indecisive, stuck, or simply dreading a writing task, that you will open this book. You will be greeted by people who understand how you feel and we will offer a few tips and tricks that have worked for us. Give some of these methods a try and you may find the writing process becomes easier for you, moves a little quicker, or at least becomes something you do not hate quite as much.

CONCLUSION

In this chapter, I presented five common barriers that are often cited as the reasons authors choose not to write. I have also provided five solutions that may help authors overcome these barriers. Remember that this book was not written for aspiring novelists who live and breathe to write. You may never have that level of passion for your writing. However, writing (particularly the ability to write stress-free) is a very useful skill that will pay dividends for you throughout your career.

In the chapters that follow you will get perspectives and recommendations on a host of writing topics as well as pragmatic and useful templates to get you started.

REFERENCES

Fiore, N. A. (2007). *The now habit: A strategic program for overcoming procrastination and enjoying guilt-free play*. New York, NY: TarcherPerigee.

Goodson, P. (2017). *Becoming an academic writer: 50 exercises for paced, productive, and powerful writing* (2nd ed.). Thousand Oaks, CA: SAGE Publications.

King, S. (2002). *On writing: A memoir of the craft*. New York, NY: Simon & Schuster.

Lamott, A. (1995). *Bird by bird*. New York, NY: Anchor Books.

Silvia, P. J. (2007). *How to write a lot: A practical guide to productive academic writing*. Washington, DC: American Psychological Association.

CHAPTER ②

WHY DO WE (HAVE TO) WRITE?

Robert Topp

PERSONAL STORY

My First "Success" in Scholarly Writing

> You really need to submit this paper to a journal for publication! Your score is 93 out of 100 points on this assignment.

This is what my instructor wrote across my final paper in my master's course titled "Introduction to Nursing Theories N601." I was ecstatic! My first 12 weeks in graduate education was paying off already. My instructor recognized what I had known all semester long: that I was a "wunderkind" and my manuscript was the breakthrough in unifying theoretical concepts to direct nursing practice. I thought every nursing student, faculty, and practicing nurse needed to read my manuscript. I immediately retyped the document without incorporating any of the "minor" revisions recommended by my instructor (why mess with perfection?) and mailed a copy to the editor of the journal, *Nursing Research*. Two weeks later I received a sky-blue envelope from the journal. Although the guidelines to authors indicated that the review process would take 3 to 4 months, I assumed the editor immediately recognized the scientific merit of my work and was fast-tracking my manuscript for the earliest possible print date. You can probably guess the content of the letter inside of the envelope. Although I did not keep this letter, I am sure it included phrases like ". . . a worthy effort," "please review the instructions to authors . . .," and "your manuscript is not suitable for further consideration." I was devastated. How could I have been so wrong? Did my instructor and the editor collude in some sadistic rite of initiation into scholarly writing in nursing? Is this an example of the nursing profession "eating their young?" After 35 years of reflecting on this seminal moment in my professional life I now realize that many nurses experience a similar epiphany when writing. This chapter is to help minimize the number of times you have similar experiences in your pursuits of scholarly writing.

INTRODUCTION

The first section of this chapter explores the reasons why nurses often do not write well, which contributes to some nurses "hating" to write or choosing not to write at all. The second section explores reasons why nurses *should* write. Finally, I explain the structure of scholarly writing and use an example of a class assignment to demonstrate how to develop the structure of a scholarly manuscript. This final section includes some general tips to help you structure a piece of writing for ease of comprehension and maximum effect.

WHY NURSES DO NOT WRITE ~~GOOD~~ WELL

> **WRITING TIP**
>
> Avoid the word "should" in scholarly writing. The use of this term implies a moral position or an opinion that the reader may not share. Instead support the statement from the literature.

Nurses are among the most passionate and dedicated health professionals I have ever encountered. When nurses apply themselves to a task, they can accomplish more in less time than any other group of professionals. So why is it that some nurses do not write well? The easy answer is they "do not apply themselves to the task" or they do not "appreciate the importance of writing." These, like most easy answers, contain only a grain of truth. Many of my students, friends, and colleagues want to write more. They spend countless hours trying to write, struggling with each keystroke. I have observed nursing students as well as junior and senior faculty members spend countless hours trying to write, achieving only average-quality results. I have observed nurses working in clinical areas struggle for weeks to write a scholarly abstract or develop the content for an evidence-based poster. I have also watched academic and clinical nurses become visibly anxious and even physically sick when just considering the task of developing a manuscript for publication. Finally, a significant proportion of doctorally prepared nursing faculty exert Herculean efforts in writing but produce relatively few scholarly written works. There are myriad reasons why many nurses avoid scholarly writing or, when they do write, struggle to produce a high-quality scholarly document.

Nursing is relatively new to the academe "scene" with the location for training nurses shifting from hospitals to universities during the 1990s (Rolfe, 2009). This transition has required nursing faculty, or "academic nurses," to be not only outstanding clinical instructors but also to adopt the values and behaviors of faculty members in other disciplines within universities. One of the hallmark expectations of university faculty members is to produce and disseminate new knowledge through scholarly writing. In other words, university faculty (including academic nurses) are expected to "publish or perish." Nursing scholarly writing has been defined as "writing that is specialized in the discipline of nursing, communicates original thought, includes support from a body of literature, contains formal language consistent with the discipline of nursing, and is formatted in a manner consistent with peer-reviewed publications" (Gazza, Shellenbarger, & Hunker, 2013). This definition of scholarly writing is not limited to publications in research and practice journals but also includes abstracts as well as articles in the popular press including newspapers, magazines, blogs, and more. A major challenge for nursing faculty has been, and continues to be, to engage in more scholarly writing when they have had limited formal training and experience with scholarly writing.

A second challenge with transitioning nursing education into universities is that a significant proportion of nursing faculty members are dedicated (almost exclusively) to educating students on clinical nursing skills. Developing clinical skills requires the consumption of scholarly writing, but documenting clinical skills does not include scholarly writing. Clinical skills are documented by listing activities, charting on forms, documenting unexpected findings, or "charting by exception." Nursing faculty who teach clinical skills rarely have the opportunity to develop learning experiences for their students that require scholarly writing or to engage in scholarly writing as a component of their academic role. A third challenge confronting nursing faculty in many universities is that their job description and workload deemphasize scholarly writing. The workload among nursing faculty in "teaching-intensive" universities often focuses on producing excellent clinical nurses with limited expectations to engage in scholarly writing. Scholarly writing skills, like any skill, deteriorate with disuse.

Whitehead (2002) concluded that graduate nursing students struggle with scholarly writing because they have limited experience with this skill. Often, there is a lack of emphasis in their program in teaching this skill and scholarly writing has not been a component of their clinical practice. The shift in nurse training into universities and the increased emphasis on evidence-based practice requires the nursing curriculum to include more assignments that involve scholarly writing. Undergraduate nursing students are required to be competent consumers of scholarly writing and to incorporate scholarly writing as evidence on which to base their practice. Graduate level nursing students are required to produce scholarly writing that generates new knowledge (e.g., PhD dissertation) or is aimed at improving nursing practice (master's degree capstone; doctor of nursing practice [DNP] projects). The challenge to many undergraduate and graduate nursing students is that most nursing programs place limited emphasis on developing scholarly writing skills in their curricula (Borglin &

Fagerström, 2012; Gazza et al., 2013). Scholarly writing has been referred to as a "game with a bewildering set of rules, many of which are never made explicit to student writers" (Harwood & Hadley, 2004).

The absence of scholarly writing within most clinical nurses' practice contributes to the "disconnect" between what is taught in nursing programs and what is expected in nursing practice (Burns & Poster, 2008). The academic progression of nurses commonly involves a "break to obtain clinical experience" before pursuing an advanced graduate degree. This is in contrast to other academic disciplines that encourage students to complete undergraduate through postdoctoral training without interruption, allowing students to develop and maintain their discipline-specific writing skills. Meanwhile, nurses frequently enter graduate programs with poor writing skills attributable to disuse.

A final explanation as to why nurses (among many others) do not write well can be attributed to a general decrease in expectation for formal writing skills. Written communication has undergone rapid transformations over the past 30 years. Advancements in technology (text messaging, social media, email, blogs, Snapchat, etc.) have changed the way people communicate through writing. Technology has led to the introduction of new words (e.g., google, tweet) and abbreviations (e.g., FAQ, LOL, TY, THX, TTYL) and the regular use of symbols (☺, :0, :P) in everyday written communication. However, these changes have had little impact on the long-accepted format and structure of scholarly writing. Publishers, editors, reviewers, and authors have not incorporated these new or hybrid forms of written communication into formal scholarly writing.

WHY NURSES NEED TO WRITE ~~MORE~~

> **WRITING TIP**
> Avoid using the terms "physician" and "doctor" interchangeably. Physicians have a medical degree and practice medicine. Doctors have a terminal academic degree in a specific discipline and are trained in the development and dissemination of knowledge.

I have been around nurses my entire professional career and I have learned that nurses have a lot to say and they say a lot. Nurses from all areas of our profession have innovative ideas for improving patient care, teaching students, and conducting research. For example, I worked with a team of clinical nurses to solve the seemingly intractable problem of cancellation of specialty cardiac procedures. The cancellation rate for procedures in the unit was 18% and the unit administrator was considering nursing staff cuts to accommodate the lost opportunity costs. "If the unit is handling 18% fewer cases, then we need to cut staff by 18%," was the administrator's position, which was supported by "the data." Our team researched the reasons why procedures were cancelled and discovered more than 30 different explanations ranging from no preprocedure EKG or blood tests, no signed consent to patients, or medical staff forgetting the time of the procedure. Thus, "the data" did not indicate an easy fix to resolving the problem of the high rate of cancellations. During a meeting with the nursing staff from this unit, an "experienced" hospital program–prepared nurse commented, "Why don't we generate a checklist for all of the reasons cases are cancelled to be completed by our staff the night before? This would allow the nursing staff to address any issues before the patient arrives for the procedure." Genius! Our team developed the checklist, including standing physician orders, for the most common issues contributing to cancellations completed by the unit staff the day before the procedure. After 3 months, "the data" indicated the cancellation rate for procedures in this unit had dropped to 4%, gross revenues increased over $200,000 at a cost of $2,000 of additional staff time per month! Despite much encouragement from me, the nurses in this clinical unit who conducted the project never published or communicated these findings beyond their unit.

This example is typical of the outstanding innovations in patient care that nurses frequently develop but never communicate through scholarly writing. Unfortunately, most nurses, for the reasons stated previously, do not write about their inventive advances in clinical practice or academic innovations. As all nurses know, if an action is not documented, then the action never took place. Our profession needs to capitalize on the frequently quoted fact that nurses have consistently been ranked as the profession with the highest honesty and ethical standards for over 15 years (Norman, 2016). Pamela F. Cipriano, PhD, RN, NEA-BC, FAAN, president of the American Nurses Association, encourages nurses to draw on this public trust of the profession of nursing to engage with consumers to improve their health. An important medium through which nurses can engage with other healthcare professionals and consumers is scholarly writing. Thus, nurses need to write about their clinical and academic improvements because the public's trust in the nursing profession legitimizes the content of the writing and nursing innovation contributes to improvement in the public health.

Other groups of nurses have additional motivations to engage in more scholarly writing. Academic nurses are expected to engage in the development and dissemination of knowledge through scholarly writing. Scholarly writing in the form of peer-reviewed manuscripts and abstracts are considered the "currency" of the university. An important metric in determining academic appointments, promotion, and tenure is the number and quality of scholarly writing productivity. Other groups of nonacademic nurses employed in the clinical setting are being asked to participate more in scholarly writing. Hospitals pursuing Magnet® status strive to include the nursing staff in developing evidence-based nursing practice policies and procedures. This process encourages clinical nurses to publish the evidence-based changes in nursing practice through scholarly writing.

In addition to scholarly writing being a requirement of specific nursing job roles, developing scholarly writing skills has a number of other advantages. Scholarly writing has the potential to change people's attitudes, their health behavior, and their lives. The pen has always been mightier than the sword (Bulwer-Lytton, 1839). Changes in nursing clinical practice and healthcare policies rely on the rationale of empirical data communicated through scholarly writing rather than on historical precedent ("the way we've always done it"). Therefore, if you wish to make a change in nursing practice or healthcare policy, the most effective mechanism is through scholarly writing. W. Edwards Deming's quote "In God we trust: all others bring data" is appropriate when attempting to effect a change in healthcare. Scholarly writing can communicate data measurement and analysis, which are essential to attaining superior performance. Another less altruistic reason to engage in scholarly writing is discipline-specific fame and fortune. It is true, there are very few groupies who follow or form fan clubs for scholarly writers. To be recognized as an authority in a particular field, you need to have produced a critical mass of scholarly manuscripts in that area. Publishing scholarly manuscripts builds your credibility as an authority in the content area of the manuscript. If you publish scholarly manuscripts, you will be sought after to assist in writing other scholarly manuscripts in exchange for authorship and other compensation. Individuals who publish scholarly manuscripts in a particular area are recognized as experts in that area and are sought after for their consultation expertise for compensation. Beyond work requirements, engaging in scholarly writing is a way of earning recognition from your peers and compensation for your expertise in the content area in which you are an author.

As we have shown you in this section, there are a number of reasons nurses need to engage in more scholarly writing. The public trusts nurses and this trust provides nurses with the platform to communicate health information through scholarly writing. Scholarly writing is the primary medium through which new knowledge is communicated in academic and clinical settings. Academic nurses who engage in scholarly writing are more likely to be promoted and receive tenure. Similarly, clinical nursing has begun to rely on scholarly writing not only for nurses' advancement but also for providing a sound basis for decisions to change clinical practice and policies within healthcare institutions. Finally, nurses who engage in scholarly writing are viewed as authorities in the content area they write about and are compensated for sharing their content expertise as well as their capacity to write.

THE STRUCTURE OF SCHOLARLY WRITING

You are probably wondering when I was going to get around to telling you something that you can actually use. So far, this chapter has talked about why nurses do not write and reasons why nurses need to write more. The next section of this chapter provides you with an overview of the general structure of scholarly writing. The structure I present includes an introduction, logical progression of content, and a conclusion. I conclude this chapter with an example of how to use this structure to write a scholarly manuscript using a college assignment as an example.

> A story must have a beginning, middle and end united by causal relationship. (Heracles by Euripides, 416 BC)

WRITING TIP

The primary purpose of scholarly writing is to communicate new knowledge. If you want to write to entertain your reader, write a mystery novel. If you want to be creative in your writing, compose haiku.

The structure of writing has not changed much since ancient Greece. To paraphrase Euripides, your writing must first tell the reader what you are going to tell them, tell the reader the relevant information, and then tell the reader what you just told them, all of which is united around a common theme. This structure permeates many different types of written communication. Have you ever wondered why most daily comic strips include three to four frames instead of two? These frames correspond roughly with the beginning, middle, and end of a story unified by a common, humorous theme. Writing is a conversation, although the author must play the part of the sender and receiver of the message. The author must anticipate how the receiver will perceive and process the message. Through written communication, the reader, or the receiver of the message, cannot ask for clarification, elaboration, or provide validation the message was received. This "asynchronous" structure of written communication places the burden of clarity on the author to introduce the message, deliver the message, and conclude the message.

To achieve the purpose of scholarly writing, communicating new knowledge, the author MUST minimize ambiguity and opportunities for alternative interpretations on the part of the reader. A successful approach to clearly communicating new knowledge is to consistently communicate the knowledge throughout a purposefully structured scholarly manuscript. Such a manuscript includes an introduction previewing the new knowledge, logically organized presentation of the content around a central theme, and a summary or review of the content that was presented.

This "beginning, middle, and end" structure is also the basis of a well-written paragraph. A paragraph communicates a single main idea. The first sentence of a paragraph provides the reader with an introduction of the overall main idea of the paragraph. The last sentence provides the reader with a summation of the content of the paragraph. The sentences between the first and last sentences of a paragraph are the content united around a common theme or main idea. Exhibit 2.1 provides an example of a well-written paragraph. The first sentence in this example explains to the reader that the content of the paragraph will include how improvements in early diagnosis and treatment of breast cancer has improved over the past two decades. The middle four sentences provide content consistent with and in support of this first sentence. Notice how the author has not cited statistics beyond the two-decade window; rather, the author only cited statistics about breast cancer as mentioned in the first sentence. The final sentence of the paragraph summarizes the content of the paragraph and is very similar in content to the first sentence in the paragraph.

EXHIBIT 2.1: PARAGRAPH EXAMPLE

[**beginning sentence**] Early diagnosis and effective treatment of breast cancer over the past two decades has improved.
[**middle sentences**] Crude, relative, and corrected 5-year survival rates have been reported to be 73%, 91%, and 82%, respectively. According to the latest estimates, cumulative 40-year relative survival is now approximately 43% for stages I-IV breast cancers, 57% for localized breast tumors, and 24% for breast cancers with regional tumor spread. In the United States, 5-year survival following breast cancer diagnosis has increased from 75% during 1974 to 1976 to 87% during 1992 to 1995. Ten-year relative survival risk currently ranges from 39% among women over age 75 to 56% among those aged 40 to 44 and 50% among patients younger than 35.
[**ending sentence**] Thus, a substantial number of patients who are initially diagnosed with breast cancer survive the disease as a result of effective treatment.

The Beginning

The initial section of a scholarly manuscript, also termed the introduction, is the most critical structural component of the document. The introduction section explains to the reader why the content is being presented (the "hook"); what the overall aim of the manuscript is (the purpose); and how the content will be presented (the structure). After reading a well-written introduction, the reader will be able to answer three questions. First, why is the author writing the manuscript? Second, what is the purpose, objective, or aim of the manuscript? In other words, what increases in knowledge will the reader realize from reading the manuscript? Finally, how will the content of the manuscript be structured to achieve the purpose? An introduction that addresses these three areas provides the reader with insight into not only why the new knowledge is important, but also how the content of the new knowledge will be presented.

The first section of a scholarly manuscript needs to "hook" the reader's interest and explain why the content or new knowledge is being presented (Exhibit 2.2). This "hook" is also termed the "problem statement," which explains to the reader some undesirable phenomenon or problem in need of being fixed. When describing this "opportunity," the author commonly includes two categories of facts or rationales that describe the scope and significance of the problem. The scope of a problem is expressed as the number of individuals affected by the undesirable phenomenon. When discussing the scope, the author can also provide insight into the population who will be the focus of the remainder of the manuscript, including species, gender, age, and any other defining characteristics. The second component of the "hook" is the significance or impact of the problem. Significance of a problem is commonly expressed in terms of three features: money, morbidity or mortality, and/or quality of life. These three features of a problem are usually interrelated. If a phenomenon degrades quality of life, then it likely increases morbidity and/or mortality and cost or wastes money. If a problem does not cost excessive amounts of money, result in sickness and/or death, or depreciate someone's ability to realize their fullest potential, then the reader will likely wonder why this new knowledge is important. Another way of thinking about the "hook" is this: If you cannot get the reader immediately interested in the potential impact of the new knowledge, he or she will not read any further.

EXHIBIT 2.2: EXAMPLES OF "HOOK" SECTIONS

Example 1

In Europe, 6% to 27% of all ICU patients die in the ICU, and in the United States 10% to 29% die [Capuzzo et al., 2014; Society of Critical Care Medicine, 2015]. In the Netherlands, nearly 8% die [one reference]. Over 85% of those deaths occur after withholding or withdrawal of life-sustaining treatment [one reference]. With the ageing population, the increasing complexity of ICU patients, and the increasing number of critically ill patients, the number of decisions to withhold or withdraw life-sustaining treatment will grow as well [Nationale IC Evaluatie, 2013]. The care provided before, during and after withholding or withdrawing life-sustaining treatment is referred to as end-of-life care (EOLC; Noome, Beneken Genaamd Kolmer, Leeuwen, Dijkstra, & Vloet, 2016).

Example 2

Childhood obesity affects 16.9% of children in the United States, with an additional 14.9% being overweight [Ogden, Carroll, Kit, & Flegal, 2014]. Children from racial minority groups and low-income households are disproportionately affected [Ogden et al., 2014; Wan & Lim, 2012]. Childhood obesity is associated with morbidity, premature mortality [Reilly & Kelly, 2011], and obesity in adulthood [Guo & Chumlea, 1999; Freedman et al., 2005]. As a result, decreasing childhood obesity is a national [U.S. Department of Health & Human Services, 2014] and global [World Health Organization, 2012] priority (Schroeder, Travers, & Smaldone, 2016).

Once your reader understands the potential impact of the new knowledge being presented in the manuscript, you can then explain the overall aim or purpose of the manuscript. While the introduction is the most critical component of your scholarly work, the purpose statement is the most critical sentence of your entire manuscript. It is commonly overtly stated as "The purpose (aim, objective) of this manuscript is to disclose, describe. . ." (see Exhibit 2.3). The purpose explains the new knowledge the will reader realize from reading the scholarly manuscript. If the manuscript is a data-based research article, then the purpose commonly includes the variables being studied, the population, and how the variables are being addressed. Variables can be described, relationships between variables can be identified, and variables affecting other variables can be detected. If the manuscript is not a data-based article, then the purpose discloses the new knowledge that will be presented.

EXHIBIT 2.3: EXAMPLES OF PURPOSE STATEMENTS

Data-Based Manuscripts

The purpose of this study was to determine whether the safety climate and the nurse's work environment make comparable or distinct contributions to patient outcomes (Olds, Aiken, Cimiotti, & Lake, 2017).

The purpose of this research was to determine if weekend and holiday presentation is associated with increased mortality in EDs among patients with acute myocardial infarction in New Jersey (de Cordova, Johansen, Martinez, & Cimiotti, 2017).

Non-Data-Based Manuscripts

A case study presented here describes a patient with muscular dystrophy who received intratympanic gentamicin (ITG) to manage intractable vertigo (Pullen, 2017).

This Western Journal of Nursing Research (WJNR) *Editorial Board Special Article addresses strategies to enhance authorship skills among PhD students* (Conn et al., 2017).

Following the purpose statement, the introduction then explains how the manuscript will be structured and the content of the work. Presentation of the structure and content of the manuscript explains to the reader how the purpose will be achieved. The content and structure of a data-based manuscript is commonly prescribed by the publishing journal and may include the following sections: background, methodology, results, discussion, and conclusion. The structure of a data-based manuscript is directed at addressing hypotheses or research questions. The content and structure of a non-data-based manuscript is more

WRITING TIP

Be consistent in stating the purpose of a manuscript. Use the cut-and-paste option when restating the purpose in a manuscript. A change in <u>any</u> words or ordering of words in a purpose statement indicates either a different purpose or a lack of attention to detail by the author.

flexible and provides the reader with an outline of how the new knowledge will be ordered in the remainder of the manuscript. This order describes the logical presentation that begins with mentioning established knowledge on which the presentation of new knowledge is built. This section also introduces the reader to definitions of terms and acronyms that will be used throughout the remainder of the manuscript. It is critical that you use the exact same terms when referring to the same concepts throughout the manuscript. For example, using the terms "older adult," "elderly," "aged," "senior citizen," interchangeably in a single scholarly manuscript would likely confuse the reader who expects a single term be used to refer to a single concept. The use of different terms implies you are referring to different concepts. Once a term is established and defined, only use that term when referring to the concept throughout your entire manuscript. When defining a term, you may need to mention all the other similar terms, which are commonly used to refer to the concept. An example of defining a term and including all related terms in the definition is as follows: "Older adults, also referred to as 'elderly,' 'aged,' or 'senior citizens' in the literature, is anyone age 65 year or older." Consistent use of terminology throughout a manuscript is a hallmark characteristic of meritorious scholarly writing.

The Middle

After reading the introduction section to a scholarly manuscript the reader has a clear idea of why, what, and how the content of the middle section of the manuscript will be delivered and the order in which it will be presented. If the manuscript is data based, then the structure commonly adheres to a uniform format dictated by the journal and described in the "Information for Authors" instructions. The introduction may also include definitions of terms and acronyms. In a scholarly manuscript that is not data based, the content in the middle section is presented in the same order as it is announced in the introduction section of the manuscript. This consistency in ordering the content between the introduction and the middle section of the manuscript minimizes the confusion the reader may experience as a result of having the content outlined in the introduction and then presented in a different order in the middle section. Another technique to help the reader identify the consistency between the introduction and the middle section is in using major and minor headings. Each of the content areas mentioned in the introduction can be used as a heading for separate sections in the middle section of the manuscript. In data-based manuscripts the content headers are often prescribed by the publishing journal and may include background, methodology, results, discussion, and conclusion. The headers in the middle section of a non-data-based manuscript need to be consistent with the topical areas the author states in the introduction. For example, if the author writes, "The purpose of this manuscript will be addressed in four sections. . .," then the author needs to have four major headings in the manuscript. Having three or five major heading in the manuscript following this purpose statement will confuse readers since they will be anticipating four separate sections. Headers in the middle section not only provide consistency with the introduction but also indicate to the reader that the content of the manuscript is progressing and is will be different from the previous section. Thus, the middle section of a manuscript closely follows the content and structure outlined in the introduction.

The End

The final section of a scholarly manuscript consists of a brief review of the content that was presented in the middle section. "The End" of a manuscript may be labeled as "Conclusion" or "Summary." The length and content of this section is similar to the introduction. The author typically restates the "hook" or the problem the manuscript addressed. "The End" reiterates the content, again, in the same order as both the introduction and the middle section. Finally, "The End" makes a concluding statement about the purpose of the manuscript. This statement clearly explains to the reader how the information they just read has achieved the purpose of the manuscript.

MINI CLASS: HOW TO WRITE A BETTER COLLEGE PAPER

This final section of this chapter demonstrates how to use the knowledge you have gained to write a scholarly paper for a college course. Papers are different from manuscripts since composing a scholarly paper is to achieve a learning objective in a course. The purpose of writing a scholarly manuscript is to share new knowledge with a wider audience who can apply the new knowledge. Before showing you how to apply this knowledge, I need to inform you of the reasons scholarly papers are used as learning experiences. As well, I want to share with you some thoughts that faculty sometimes have when grading scholarly papers. These reasons for assigning scholarly papers and faculty thoughts when grading these assignments are NOT universal truths but may help you to understand the audience for whom you are writing and why you are writing for them.

Contrary to what you may believe, scholarly papers are not assigned as a way of torturing students, developing a difficult course, or vetting weaker students from academically intense or competitive programs. Faculty assign scholarly papers as learning experiences for several reasons. Learning objectives achieved through a student composing a scholarly paper commonly involve demonstrating higher levels of knowledge integration and/or cognitive processing (Anderson et al., 2001). Composing a scholarly paper requires you to not only have read and retained the knowledge (at least through the completion of the paper) but also requires you to apply or describe the knowledge in some new way. The knowledge in a scholarly paper composed as a course assignment may not be new, but the application or combination of the knowledge needs to be novel. This new application of established knowledge indicates you have a greater integration, processing, and utilization of the knowledge. Composing a scholarly paper also provides the instructor with insight into your understanding of the content. If your manuscript clearly and logically presents content, this shows the instructor that you have a clear comprehension and understanding of the information. Similarly, composing a scholarly paper encourages you to follow instructions and work within deadlines. Composing a scholarly paper requires revisions, discipline to follow instructions, and time to process the information into a coherent structure. Finally, assigning scholarly papers teaches you how to discover, integrate, and process new information in the future, prior to and following graduation without being driven to do so by a faculty's grade.

In addition to understanding the reasons why scholarly manuscripts are assigned, you also need to understand what your faculty may be thinking when grading these assignments. Understanding your audience or reader is an important consideration that will be discussed in more detail throughout this book. Box 2.1 presents some thoughts faculty may have when grading students' scholarly papers. Although these thoughts may be driven by hunger, stress, caffeine deficiency, or other demons, they provide you with a window into what faculty, at times, contemplate when grading student's scholarly papers.

BOX 2.1: THOUGHTS FACULTY MAY HAVE WHEN GRADING A SCHOLARLY MANUSCRIPT

1. Why did I wait till the last minute to grade these 30 ten-page papers? That's 300 pages I need to read and critique in the next 6 hours, or 50 pages an hour or just about one page a minute.

2. Will I get these papers graded in time to return them to the students when I said I would?

(continued)

> **BOX 2.1:** THOUGHTS FACULTY MAY HAVE WHEN GRADING A SCHOLARLY MANUSCRIPT (*continued*)
>
> 3. I have read this paragraph three times and I still have no idea what this student is trying to say.
>
> 4. I wonder how much more time I should spend editing the grammar, structure, and format of this paper?
>
> 5. Why isn't this student getting it? Did this student listen to what I said in class or read the instructions?

With this understanding, you need to make reading and evaluating your manuscript as painless as possible by incorporating the following techniques.

Tips for an A+ Scholarly Manuscript

WRITING TIP

FOLLOW THE INSTRUCTOR'S DIRECTIONS

When you do not follow the instructions, you are saying to the instructor "I know a better way of organizing this assignment; let me teach you." Or "I do not know how to follow instructions and therefore I shouldn't be in college."

First, follow the directions for the scholarly paper assignment provided by the instructor (see Exhibit 2.4 for an example of a scholarly writing assignment). The purpose of the instructions is to help you develop the structure and content of your manuscript. You need to use the words and phrases from instructions when constructing the introduction that will guide the entire manuscript. When you use the same words and phrases in your introduction that the faculty member provided in the directions, you are telling the faculty member that you have read the directions and you intend to comply. The directions inform you of the purpose and provide you with a guide to the overall content and structure of your manuscript. Well-written, detailed directions to a scholarly manuscript can even provide you with a preliminary outline of the manuscript. These well-written directions may inform you of the number of sections you need to develop and the content of those sections.

Avoid asking the faculty member to modify the directions for a written scholarly assignment. Most faculty bristle at teaching advice from students. I recall having a student tell me that it was not possible to write the content I requested in the assignment directions in 10 pages and that she needed 15 pages. I responded that by completing this assignment within the 10-page limit she would "glean the invaluable skill of parsimony, which is a prized attribute among administrators in the professional world." Other less supportive faculty might think, "T.S. (terribly sad). All my past students completed this assignment in 10 pages. Why are you special?" Creativity in interpreting the directions is rarely received positively by course faculty and your grade WILL suffer if you do not follow the directions.

Second, consistently use defined terms, acronyms, and phrases that you introduce early in the manuscript. By restating exactly the purpose, hypotheses, research questions, and so forth, you are indicating to your reader that these guiding concepts within your manuscript are not changing or "drifting" over the course of the manuscript. When you define terms early in the manuscript, the reader shares your understanding of the concept the term represents throughout the entire manuscript. The concept of consistency applies not only to terms but also to consistently applying formatting rules such as the beast that is the American Psychological Association, or APA, format. Often, this means having to adjust the default settings within your word processing program so that you do not end up with extra spaces, multiple fonts, or other unintentional alterations in format.

Third, give the reader clues in the text about the content. Use headers to identify different sections of the text that were presented in the introduction. Another technique for informing the reader about the content is providing transition sentences at the beginning of paragraphs in each new content section of the manuscript. These transitions provide "links" for the reader between different content sections in the manuscript. Transitions inform readers what they have just read and provide the linkage between this previous content and the content in the upcoming section.

Fourth, the first and final sentences of a paragraph summarize the content of a paragraph. By reading the first and last sentences and "skimming" the middle section of a paragraph, an overburdened faculty may speed-read portions of a scholarly manuscript. Summary sentences at the beginning and end of a paragraph increase the comprehension of the content among readers whose attention may be distracted while reading.

Fifth, write in third-person active tense. This style of writing uses pronouns like he, she, it, or they. This is the style of most scholarly writing in the discipline of nursing. This style will direct you toward using active instead of passive voice. Using this style will also help you avoid injecting subjective or personalized terms or affect into your text. Scholarly writing is objective and communicates empirical knowledge and facts. Including phrases like "I feel. . ." or "We believe. . ." allows the reader to interpret your content as biased, based on subjective feelings or opinions that the reader may not share. Third person is declarative and based on commonly accepted, shared perceptions and facts, which is the basis of collective knowledge.

Sixth, did I mention following the directions given to you by the instructor?

EXHIBIT 2.4: AN EXAMPLE OF A SCHOLARLY WRITING ASSIGNMENT WITH DISSECTING COMMENTARY

Directions From the Instructor:

For your final assignment in PHDN 608 Nursing Measurement, submit a **10–15 page** scholarly paper (40% of total grade) no later than **midnight on December 3 concerning the measurement of a selected health-related phenomenon.** **This paper will have two sections.** The **first section** will include a statement of rationale for the need to develop an instrument along with a critique of existing instruments to measure the chosen phenomenon and document the need to develop a new instrument or modify an established instrument(s) to measure the phenomenon. The **second section** will present a plan to develop a **new instrument or modify an established instrument(s)** to measure the selected health-related phenomenon. **This plan may include presentation** of an initial instrument and descriptions of a research project(s) to establish various forms of validity and reliability including sample(s) selection and statistical analysis.

Assignment objectives: Following completion of the assignment the student will be able to

Do not turn in a paper less than 10 or greater than 15 pages.

The manuscript is due on or before this deadline.

Explains that there are two major sections in the manuscript.

The purpose of the manuscript is to discuss the measurement of a select health-related phenomenon that the student selects.

Explains the content of the first section is the rationale for an instrument to measure a health-related phenomenon.

Explains that the second section will present a plan to develop an instrument to measure a health-related phenomenon.

The plan can include developing a new instrument or modifying an existing instrument.

Explains that this plan includes a description of the instrument and how to develop validity and reliability through conducting various research project(s).

(continued)

EXHIBIT 2.4: AN EXAMPLE OF A SCHOLARLY WRITING ASSIGNMENT WITH DISSECTING COMMENTARY (*continued*)

Through completing this scholarly paper, the instructor wants the student to be able to identify reasons that an instrument measuring a health-related phenomenon needs to be measured.

a. **Identify** the rationale for the development of an instrument to measure a select health phenomenon.

Through completing this scholarly paper, the instructor wants the student to be able to assess the benefits and limitations of existing instruments that measure some health-related phenomenon and, based on this assessment, recommend developing a new instrument or modifying an established instrument.

b. **Critique** existing instruments to measure a select health-related phenomenon and based on this critique, recommend the development of a new instrument or modification of an existing instrument.

Through completing this scholarly paper, the instructor wants the student to be able to come up with a plan to make an existing instrument better or develop a new instrument.

c. **Plan** how to develop the new instrument or modify the existing instrument to measure a select health phenomenon.

Notice how the following outline of the scholarly manuscript is consistent with the directions. The health-related phenomenon I selected as the central concept of this manuscript is sleep quality.

Outline of the Manuscript:
The First Section:

• Rationale for developing an instrument to measure sleep quality.

• Critique of existing instruments to measure sleep quality.

• Documentation for the need to develop a new instrument to measure sleep quality.

The Second Section

• Present a plan to develop a new instrument.

• Proposed methods.

• How validity and reliability will be established.

• Sample selection.

• Statistical analysis.

(continued)

EXHIBIT 2.4: AN EXAMPLE OF A SCHOLARLY WRITING ASSIGNMENT WITH DISSECTING COMMENTARY (*continued*)

[Note to reader: The intention of the following section is to provide you with an example of how to structure the content of a manuscript and NOT to provide you with the entire manuscript. Thus, the following includes only partial sections of the entire manuscript, which is intended to provide an example of the structure and NOT to communicate any scholarly content.]

Introduction

The purpose: Stated using terms similar to the directions "... measurement of a selected health phenomenon ..."

This paper will examine the measurement of the health-related phenomenon of sleep quality. Sleep quality has been defined by

Definition of the central concept of the manuscript.

When you refer to previous authors you need to provide a citation to what you are referencing.

various authors and consists of the individual's perceived

satisfaction with his or her sleep behavior (Harvey,

Stinson, Whitaker, Moskovitz, & Virk, 2008; Krystal & Edinger, 2008).

The "hook," which states the scope and significance of the problem of declining sleep quality in older adults.

Up to 80% of adults age 65 years and older report declines

A definition of the term "older adult."

in their sleep quality. Poor sleep quality reported by older

adults predicts a variety of comorbidities including cognitive

decline (Yaffe, Falvey, & Hoang, 2014), falls (Stone et al., 2014), and

cardiovascular disease (Foley, Ancoli-Israel, Britz, & Walsh, 2004).

Statements of how the content will be structured in the middle section of the manuscript. Notice how the structure, with two main sections and multiple topical areas within these two sections are consistent with the directions. This consistency tells the instructor that you are going to structure the manuscript consistent with ther instructions.

Measurement of sleep quality among older adults will be

explored in two sections in this paper. The first section includes

rationale for developing an instrument to measure sleep

quality. Following the presentation of this rationale, a critique

of existing instruments to measure sleep quality is offered.

Finally, this first section provides documentation for the need to develop a

(*continued*)

EXHIBIT 2.4: AN EXAMPLE OF A SCHOLARLY WRITING ASSIGNMENT WITH DISSECTING COMMENTARY (*continued*)

new instrument to measure sleep quality. Following this, the second section of this paper presents a plan to develop a new instrument to measure sleep quality among older adults. This plan includes a description of proposed methods to establish various forms of validity and reliability including sample selection and statistical analysis.

I. **How Sleep Quality is Measured**

a. Sleep Quality in Older Adults

Introductory sentence indicates that this subsection will be discussing how poor sleep quality affects the biological, psychological, and social functioning of older adults.

Poor sleep quality or the individual's perceived satisfaction with his or her sleep behavior negatively effects the bio/psycho/social functioning of older adults.

b. Existing Measures of Sleep Quality

Notice the transition sentence to help the reader recognize a new content section is starting and how this new content is linked with the previous section.

Since sleep quality has been demonstrated to have a negative impact on many aspects of functioning among older adults, a number of measures have been developed to quantify sleep quality. The literature includes a number of measures of sleep quality that are described and critiqued including the Pittsburg Sleep Quality Index, actigraphy, and EEG recordings.

This sentence provides an outline for this section that the these three measures of sleep quality are going to be critiqued.

c. Limitations in Measuring Sleep Quality

Although the three measures of sleep quality reviewed in the previous section are widely used to measure sleep quality, each of them exhibits limitation in the measurement of this concept.

Notice the transition guiding the reader from the description of the three measures to a discussion of the limitations of each measure. This presentation of the limitations of each measurement will provide the justification for developing a new measure.

d. Conclusion of How Sleep Is Measured

Older adults experience declines in their sleep quality that is correlated with declines in functioning. The three most common measures of sleep quality among older adults, including the Pittsburg Sleep Quality Index, actigraphy, and EEG recordings, each has limitations. The next section of this paper describes development of a new measure of sleep quality to address the limitations of these established instruments.

Notice how this paragraph summarizes the first section of the paper and provides rationale for the second section. That is telling readers what they just read and how it is related to what they are about to read.

(*continued*)

EXHIBIT 2.4: AN EXAMPLE OF A SCHOLARLY WRITING ASSIGNMENT WITH DISSECTING COMMENTARY (*continued*)

II.   **Developing a New Measure of Sleep Quality**

   a.   Research plan

This is the introduction to the second section of the paper. Notice the consistent use and ordering of terms and phrases from the introduction. After reading this, the reader clearly understands the upcoming content and order of that content.

This section describes a plan of a research study to develop a new instrument to measure sleep quality among older adults. This plan describes the study methodology to establish validity and reliability of this new instrument including study design, sample selection, instrument item development, and a statistical analysis plan. The research design is a series of descriptive studies first to establish the face and content validity of the new instrument followed by additional studies to establish internal consistency and test–rest reliability . . .

   ○   Design

   ○   Sample

   ○   Development of Sleep Quality Items on the Measure

   ○   Procedure

   b.   Establishing Validity and Reliability

   c.   Statistical Analysis Plan

   d.   Conclusion of Developing a New Measure

The conclusion of the paper is very similar to the introduction. The conclusion states how the purpose of the paper was achieved by reviewing the content of the paper in the order in which it was presented.

Keep telling the instructor that you followed the directions.

Conclusion

This paper has examined the measurement of the health-related phenomenon of sleep quality among older adults. This purpose was addressed in two sections. The first section described how

Tell the instructor you followed the directions.

the problem of declining sleep quality among older adults is related to declines in functioning. Next, three common measures of sleep quality were described including the limitations of each of these measures. These limitations provided the rationale for developing a new measure of sleep quality among older adults. The second section of this paper described a research plan to develop a new measure of sleep quality. This plan described the methodologies of a number of studies that would establish the validity and reliability of this new measure of sleep quality among older adults.

CONCLUSION

After reading this chapter you hopefully have a better idea of why nurses do not engage in scholarly writing. I also made a strong case in this chapter for why nurses need to participate in more scholarly writing. The initial part of the chapter laid the foundation for the second section of the chapter. In the second section, I gave you an overview of the general structure of scholarly writing. This overview described the structure and content of the three sections of a scholarly manuscript including the beginning, the middle, and the end. I then demonstrated how to use this structure when writing a scholarly paper for a college course. This demonstration presented the instructor's directions for the paper, a brief outline, and partial sections of the entire paper. Within each of these sections I dissected the content to describe the rationale for the structure and the content.

This chapter, which describes the structure and content of scholarly writing, provides the foundation for the remaining sections of the book.

REFERENCES

Anderson, L. W., Krathwohl, D. R., Airasian, P., Cruikshank, K., Mayer, R., Pintrich, P., . . . Wittrock, M. (2001). *A taxonomy for learning, teaching and assessing: A revision of Bloom's taxonomy*. New York, NY: Longman Publishing.

Borglin, G., & Fagerström, C. (2012). Nursing students' understanding of critical thinking and appraisal and academic writing: A descriptive, qualitative study. *Nurse Education in Practice, 12*(6), 356–360. doi:10.1016/j.nepr.2012.04.009

Bulwer-Lytton, E. (1839). *Richelieu; or, the conspiracy: A play in five acts*. New York, NY: Harper and Brothers.

Burns, P., & Poster, E. C. (2008). Competency development in new registered nurse graduates: Closing the gap between education and practice. *Journal of Continuing Education in Nursing, 39*(2), 67–73.

Conn, V. S., Jefferson, U., Cohen, M. Z., Anderson, C. M., Killion, C. M., Fahrenwald, N. L., . . . Smith, C. E. (2017). *Strategies to build authorship competence among PhD students*. Thousand Oaks, CA: SAGE Publications.

de Cordova, P. B., Johansen, M. L., Martinez, M. E., & Cimiotti, J. P. (2017). Emergency department weekend presentation and mortality in patients with acute myocardial infarction. *Nursing Research, 66*(1), 20–27. doi:10.1097/NNR.0000000000000196

Foley, D., Ancoli-Israel, S., Britz, P., & Walsh, J. (2004). Sleep disturbances and chronic disease in older adults: Results of the 2003 National Sleep Foundation Sleep in America Survey. *Journal of Psychosomatic Research, 56*(5), 497–502. doi:10.1016/j.jpsychores.2004.02.010

Gazza, E. A., Shellenbarger, T., & Hunker, D. F. (2013). Developing as a scholarly writer: The experience of students enrolled in a PhD nursing program in the United States. *Nurse Education Today, 33*(3), 268–274. doi:10.1016/j.nedt.2012.04.019

Harvey, A. G., Stinson, K., Whitaker, K. L., Moskovitz, D., & Virk, H. (2008). The subjective meaning of sleep quality: A comparison of individuals with and without insomnia. *Sleep, 31*(3), 383–393.

Harwood, N., & Hadley, G. (2004). Demystifying institutional practices: Critical pragmatism and the teaching of academic writing. *English for Specific Purposes, 23*(4), 355–377. doi:10.1016/j.esp.2003.08.001

Krystal, A. D., & Edinger, J. D. (2008). Measuring sleep quality. *Sleep medicine, 9*, S10–S17. doi:10.1016/S1389-9457(08)70011-X

Noome, M., Beneken Genaamd Kolmer, D. M., Leeuwen, E., Dijkstra, B. M., & Vloet, L. C. M. (2016). The role of ICU nurses in the spiritual aspects of end-of-life care in the ICU: An explorative study. *Scandinavian Journal of Caring Sciences, 31*(3), 569–578.

Norman, J. (2016). *Americans rate health care providers high on honesty, ethics.* Washington, DC: Gallup Inc.

Olds, D. M., Aiken, L. H., Cimiotti, J. P., & Lake, E. T. (2017). Association of nurse work environment and safety climate on patient mortality: A cross-sectional study. *International Journal of Nursing Studies, 74*, 155–161. doi: 10.1016/j.ijnurstu.2017.06.004

Pullen Jr., R. L. (2017). Navigating the challenges of Meniere disease. *Nursing, 47*(7), 38–45. doi:10.1097/01.NURSE.0000520504.06428.ce

Rolfe, G. (2009). Writing-up and writing-as: Rediscovering nursing scholarship. *Nurse Education Today, 29*(8), 816–820. doi:10.1016/j.nedt.2009.05.015

Schroeder, K., Travers, J., & Smaldone, A. (2016). Are school nurses an overlooked resource in reducing childhood obesity? A systematic review and meta-analysis. *Journal of School Health, 86*(5), 309–321. doi: 10.1111/josh.12386

Stone, K. L., Blackwell, T. L., Ancoli-Israel, S., Cauley, J. A., Redline, S., Marshall, L. M., & Ensrud, K. E. (2014). Sleep disturbances and risk of falls in older community-dwelling men: The outcomes of sleep disorders in older men (MrOS Sleep) study. *Journal of the American Geriatrics Society, 62*(2), 299–305. doi:10.1111/jgs.12649

Whitehead, D. (2002). The academic writing experiences of a group of student nurses: A phenomenological study. *Journal of Advanced Nursing, 38*(5), 498–506.

Yaffe, K., Falvey, C. M., & Hoang, T. (2014). Connections between sleep and cognition in older adults. *The Lancet Neurology, 13*(10), 1017–1028. doi:10.1016/S1474-4422(14)70172-3

CHAPTER ③

GETTING STARTED: HAVING SOMETHING TO SAY

Joseph Perazzo

PERSONAL STORY

"I cannot believe this is happening." That is all I could think as I walked to the emergency meeting I called with my dissertation chair. I was knee-deep in the data collection phase of my PhD. I was more dedicated to this work than any I had done before, spending most of my days in the lobby of a local HIV treatment center hoping to find referrals for my study. Meanwhile, I had used my time to make a lot of progress writing my dissertation. Then the unthinkable happened. Google alerts told me I should check out an article that may be of interest to me. I opened the article and my stomach dropped. Some sociopath of a scientist had published an article about his recent work, which appeared to be the exact study I was doing. I immediately wrote my chair and asked if I could stop by and that it was urgent. On the walk to her office I imagined what she would tell me: "I know this is frustrating, but you cannot copy their work. So, we need to start over." I could not have been more wrong. After she read through the article, she said, "I don't understand what you are upset about." Incredulously, I explained that I could not believe someone had done the study I was doing and that now I had to start from scratch. She looked amused and said, "I hate to break it to you, but you aren't the only one who is interested in helping people with HIV. You don't have to start over; your study is completely different, take a look." She went through the paper with me and showed me that my research questions were different, the population I was studying was different, and the direction I wanted to take with my work was different. She helped me realize that my research projects and my writing make small but significant contributions toward a better understanding of a phenomenon. I learned that what has been and is being done by others in addition to my contributions will push knowledge forward. In the end, I finished school, I published my study, and have continued to cite that wonderful sociopath in my work today.

INTRODUCTION

Anyone given the task of writing has experienced the overwhelming feeling of having nothing new to say at the very beginning. There were so many times I stared at a blank screen wondering when my fingers would start typing. Whether you are writing a paper for a class, preparing a project to climb the clinical ladder, or writing a dissertation, this can be one of the most frustrating points in the writing process. You may often engage in passionate discussions with friends, family, and coworkers about a societal health problem or patient population. However, when it comes to writing about it, you suddenly experience a debilitating case of agraphia. Does this sound familiar? When you begin to dig into the research in your area of interest, you will likely see that there is more to your topic than you ever imagined. I remember reading the work of other people with similar interests, and thinking, "Why didn't I think of that?" Or, "Darn! They got to it first!" Not to worry; the purpose of this chapter is to provide you with some tools for researching and organizing information about your topic of interest. The first two sections of this chapter discuss where good ideas for writing come from, and how to go from asking questions to knowing a topic well enough to write about it. In the third section of this chapter, I discuss the importance of reviewing scientific literature. I present two tools that will help you organize background research in a way that will set you up for successful writing and provide you with simple templates for each. Now let's start get started!

WHERE GOOD IDEAS FOR WRITING COME FROM

There are few things I know with *complete* certainty—one is that the work of nurses is very important, another is that a lot of people, including those who are not nurses, can benefit from a nurse's knowledge. I never tire of listening to nurses share their experiences from the bedside, in the community, or in the classroom. I had a life-changing experience when I was caring for a patient who had been hospitalized due to complications related to untreated HIV. I assumed he didn't know he was infected. I was wrong. During a conversation he said, "I wish

I had just gotten treatment when they told me I had this 4 years ago." I was stunned. Furthermore, while planning to discharge this patient, I learned that it had been a long time since he had contact with his family. His family cut ties with him when they found out that he had HIV, just days after he was diagnosed. I found myself thinking about his situation constantly; I could not imagine how difficult it must have been to learn about his diagnosis and lose his family in the same week. I began to ask a lot of the following questions:

- Why is there still so much stigma attached to HIV despite all the progress that has been made?

- Why did he wait so long to come in and get treatment? Didn't anyone call him after he tested positive and follow up?

- Was there something about the way he was told about his diagnosis that caused him to disappear from healthcare for 4 years?

- Is it normal for people to wait to get care? Is it denial or something similar?

- Did he even have any legitimate idea about what was happening to him?

As it turns out, I was not the only person who has asked these questions. Entire books have been written about HIV-related stigma. Nurses, providers, scientists, activists, and many others continue to publish books, journal articles, blogs, and contributions to the media about ways to help people living with HIV. I wanted to be part of this effort, but how? I am a clinical nurse, not an expert in this area. I soon returned to graduate school and realized that all the work I was reading began with ideas and questions and these questions were the foundation for what would become the basis for my dissertation. At first, I was upset because I thought all the good ideas had been taken but soon realized that even after all the reading I had done, I still had questions. Take a moment to think about what interests or excites you in your field. What are you passionate about? What do you think will help a certain group of individuals or society as a whole? An easy way to start is to reflect on times when you have thought or talked about your ideas using phrases like any of the following:

- "I wish they would figure out a way to. . ."
- "What bozo hatched this?"
- "If only there were something more we could do for people who. . .."
- "There has to be an easier way to. . ."
- "I do not understand why we do. . .."
- "This is the way we have always done this, but why?"

- "This policy makes things much more difficult. It would be better if we were just allowed to. . .."
- "This simply isn't working. . .."

Some of the most influential scientific ideas got their start this way and writing is often the only way to share these ideas with others. Today, nurses constantly add valuable insight and evidence to the current body of knowledge. Scholarly writing provides a crucial conduit for nurses to communicate the new knowledge they develop to the scientific community. It allows nurses to disseminate evidence to develop best practices in the clinical setting, to influence healthcare policy and decision-making, and to improve the health of communities worldwide. I sometimes hear people say that they are worried that the topics they are passionate about are not "interesting" or "exciting" enough. While I would never want to sell any nurse short, I have yet to see anyone camp outside of the nearest campus bookstore to be the first in line to buy the latest nursing theory book. I also do not know of anyone who has been injured in a stampede of rabid readers trying to be first to get the latest infection control guidelines. However, I am proud to say that nurses have been instrumental in contributing to writing these and countless other important manuscripts that have advanced healthcare.

Nurses offer a unique body of holistic knowledge grounded in years of patient care. Remember, ideas designed to generate new nursing knowledge are ideas that help very *real people* with very *real problems* to get very *real results*. If you believe in your idea, then you have everything you need to make your start! One of the hardest lessons to learn is that not everyone will like your idea or think it is important. Some people are offended when we nurses bring up the fascinating topic of wound care at the dinner table. If you begin the task of writing knowing that you are contributing something valuable through your education and experience that you want to share with others, then you cannot go wrong. The rest is patience, practice, and dedication to developing writing skills.

From Asking Questions to Generating Writing Topics

While the value of professional experience cannot be overstated, scholarly writing requires taking steps beyond one's own experience to understand the bigger picture. Personal experiences enhance understanding and often drive our efforts to learn more about a healthcare problem. It can be a difficult pill to swallow, but personal experiences alone are often insufficient to understand specific ways that problems affect or apply to diverse populations. Remember, your writing will be read by others in different environments and caring for different groups of patients. Bodies of scientific knowledge are built by the continued synthesis of information from diverse sources. Unfortunately, no one can know and do all things (except, of course, for Chuck Norris). Gaining and maintaining knowledge is an ongoing process that evolves as you are exposed to new experiences, content, and ideas. A great starting point for writing is to learn what is already known about your chosen topic from others who have investigated it. In Chapter 1, Reasons Not to Write and Getting Past them, you learned that a key component that defines scholarly writing is support from a body of literature on a given topic (Gazza, Shellenbarger, & Hunker, 2013). You can use available resources to search and review published literature, become familiar with what health organizations and authorities say about a problem, and synthesize this knowledge to find out what is known and what still needs to be done and written. Remember, talk is cheap and the written word endures. The next section provides a discussion about reviewing literature and developing your specific writing topic.

The Literature Review

The term "literature" in the context of scholarly writing primarily refers to papers that have gone through a peer review process before being published. If possible, it is helpful (and reliable) to use literature search engines through your institution and only to pull information from websites that report peer-reviewed research (e.g., the Centers for Disease Control and Prevention, the World Health Organization, the Department of Health and Human Services). Depending on your area of interest, there may be web resources dedicated to foundations and advocacy groups that also fund and publish research (e.g., the National Cancer Foundation).

Reviewing the literature on your topic can often be overwhelming due to the daunting amount of material that has already been published. It is common to feel like everyone else has taken all the good ideas. Yesterday you thought you were taking the world by storm with new knowledge and now you have enough published work on your topic that, if stacked, you could build yourself a vacation home in the country. Looking closer, the real challenge is often that the topic you are interested in (and thus, the literature review) is broad and all encompassing, instead of focused on a topic that can manageably be reviewed and written about. For example, your topic may start off as "I am interested in writing about women with breast cancer who are going through chemotherapy." This is an excellent topic! However, it is also a topic with an enormous volume of establish literature. Typing the terms "women," "breast cancer," and "chemotherapy" into Google Scholar results in over 1 million manuscript citations. If you continue pursuing the broad topic, you will quite literally be dedicating your *entire* life (and three generations after you) to reading and becoming familiar with this ever-expanding topic.

It is all too easy to become frustrated and jump to the conclusion that there is nothing left to be written on this topic. However, do not throw in the towel too early. Rather, look at how you can narrow or focus your interest in this topical area. Be more specific about your interests and compare your specific ideas to what has already been published. Look at what other scientists have to say in the discussion sections of their manuscripts about what still needs to be done. With patience and work, a more narrow or focused topic will emerge. To illustrate, here is an example of how you can take the broad topic presented previously and narrow it down to something manageable.

What specifically interests you about the process of going through chemotherapy?

- *A specific symptom, complication, or experience?*
- *An intervention?*

Initial Topic → Women with breast cancer who are going through **chemotherapy**

Narrowed Topic → The impact of exercise on women with breast cancer who are going through **chemotherapy**

Are we talking about all exercise?

More Narrowed Topic → The impact of aerobic exercise on women with breast cancer who are going through **chemotherapy**

What aspect of chemotherapy do you think exercise will help?

Even *More* Narrowed Topic → The impact of aerobic exercise on fatigue symptoms in women with breast cancer who are going through **chemotherapy**

Are you going to account for all women who go through chemotherapy?

Manageable Topic → The impact of aerobic exercise on fatigue symptoms in adult women (age ≥50 years) with breast cancer who are currently receiving chemotherapy

The rest of this chapter is dedicated to giving you some tools to help you in the process of narrowing the information you find on your topic: the running document and the literature table. I will present each of these and provide you with a guide for making your own.

The Running Document

Your running document is a document where you can constantly write down important facts, figures, impactful statements, and even random brainstorming. Check out Appendix 3.1 at the end of this chapter. You can easily do this in Microsoft Word. Use the table feature or create headings for each piece of information you want to remember for your writing. Save the file on a flash drive, in the cloud, on your computer, or all of these so that it is readily available to you. This will be a document that you can visit many times, consistently adding and updating information. Beginning your running document is simple. Consult reliable sources and begin writing down crucial information that you learn about your topic. For example, if your topic is about a disease or health condition, understanding the epidemiology of that disease will always be useful to you when you write. If you are writing about a topic that is *not* a disease (e.g., noise levels in the ICU), you will still want to know the related facts and figures that comprise that phenomenon (e.g., ICU admission statistics, science about the effect of noise on sleep). When you collect and continually revisit this information, you learn more and more about the topic and it becomes much easier to write about it. Use the following questions as a guide to learning more about your topic of interest. Bear in mind these are suggestions that are meant to be inclusive of a wide range of phenomena. You can and should modify or add to this question list.

- How many people are affected by [topic] globally? Nationally? In my state? In my city? In my county? In my hospital?
- What types of people are most affected by [topic]? (e.g., age, racial/ethnic background, socioeconomic status.)
- What are the consequences of a person encountering/catching/contending with/being exposed to/failing to [topic]?
- What treatments/solutions/strategies/resources are available to promote/treat/improve/prevent [topic]?
- What are some of the successes from current treatments/solutions/strategies/resources?
- What treatments/solutions/strategies/resources have not worked? Why?
- What types of studies/investigations/methods have been used to study [topic]?
- Is there a group/population/geographic area/healthcare setting that little is known about?
- What suggestions are made for future research about [topic]?

Unless you have total recall and can remember everything you have read at a moment's notice, your running document will be your best friend and your "second brain." It will save you countless hours repeatedly searching for references you vaguely recall. Gone will be the days of endless re-reading, teeth grinding, wall punching, and so forth because you have a user-friendly tool to help you quickly find the information you need. When you see important facts, statistics, costs, or potential solutions, add them to your document along with a reference.

The next section is dedicated to discussing how to create a complementary tool to your running document that you can use when reviewing individual research articles. First, however, I want to share some insight on this phase of the writing process. The truth is, a literature review can send you down a bottomless self-perpetuating rabbit hole. You want to be informed about your topic, but that does not mean that you must read every article that has been written about your topic before you can start writing. New articles are published every day and you will never write if you try to read them all before beginning your writing. Papers often have page or word limits, and rarely facilitate an exhaustive literature review (unless reviewing the literature is the purpose of the publication). Furthermore, the literature is always evolving. Any scientist will tell you that scientific findings are often here today and gone tomorrow as new knowledge is generated. In most cases, you want to find literature that is current (e.g., published within the last 5 to 10 years unless it is a piece of foundational work that should always be present, such as the original paper describing a measure) and relevant to your topic. Most importantly, start writing!

You do not have to have a complete running document or make sure you have reviewed every piece of published work before writing. Remember, these are tools to help you organize information to help you write, not to monopolize all your time and prevent you from writing. While I know this chapter couldn't get much more fun than I have already made it, buckle your seatbelts because now we are going to talk about reading scientific literature.

Getting Started With Your Literature Review

Now I briefly discuss a few suggestions that will hopefully make your life easier when doing a literature search.

Consult a Reference Librarian

A well-organized, narrowed Google Scholar search does not always return appropriate manuscripts. Reference librarians are skilled at navigating complex databases to help you find what is available based on the information you want to find. This is particularly helpful when your topic may be referenced in multiple ways in the literature. When authors publish papers, they are asked to provide key words; these words are intended to help other researchers locate relevant work. However, you could miss something if you search for "Exercise" instead of "Physical Activity," or "AIDS" instead of "Human Immunodeficiency Virus." Thus, if you have access to a librarian, use this resource!

Screen Titles and Abstracts

It is common for literature searches to return duplicate citations and off-topic citations. It is important to screen the titles and abstracts of articles to determine whether they are appropriate for the topic on which you are writing. While much may have been written on a topic, no one expects you to look up and read 16,550 articles for the manuscript you are writing.

Read Published Literature Reviews

Journals will publish literature reviews, particularly when many authors have written about an important topic. Published literature reviews can help you find new references in addition to your own search and may even provide you with new insight into your topic. It is important that you do not take any one interpretation of the literature as accurate; always access the original source when citing that source.

Imagine that you now have a manageable, and often large, collection of articles on your topic. Many scholars have recommend creating a literature review table (Appendix 3.2; sometimes called a literature review matrix) to help you organize your literature search (Garrard, 2016; Melnyk & Morrison-Beedy, 2012). A table provides you with the ability to document and synthesize many articles in a compact and succinct way, focusing only on the most relevant content of the article. Remember, reviewing scientific literature is not the same thing as reading fictional mysteries and thrillers. Few scholarly manuscripts are written to be entertaining and not every author can captivate their readers. Rather, scholarly manuscripts are structured to pull crucial information from them. As you continue to read more on your topic, you will begin to see prominent scientists' names repeatedly and will become more and more familiar with background information. Organization is key. Anyone who writes regularly will agree there is nothing more maddening than furiously flipping or scrolling through dozens of manuscripts trying to find that one fact you *know* is out there and that you need to reference.

You can use a number of software programs to create your table (e.g., Microsoft Word, Microsoft Excel)—any software that allows you to make a series of rows and columns. While you may want to create various tables that collect different types of information about a topic, a good place to start is to collect the following information for your table:

- Who wrote the article and what year was it published?
- What was the purpose of the study/literature review/article?
- What were the characteristics of the sample?
- What was the intervention investigated?
- What were the results of the study?
- How does this study contribute to what you are interested in? What do the authors recommend for future research? What was NOT done in this study?

Remember, do not fall into "analysis paralysis." You do not have to review all the literature before you begin to write. In an example paragraph at the end of this chapter, I show you how I formed an introductory paragraph with current (at the time) data. Getting my writing started did not require an exhaustive literature review.

I have one last piece of advice about reviewing literature. When I was a student, I (like many) seemed to never heed the professor's warning not to wait until the last minute to begin writing an assignment. Creating a table and reviewing literature is much easier to do incrementally than in a weekend binge. If you can choose a number of manuscripts you will read per day, perhaps first thing in the morning or before you go to bed (and some manuscripts rival melatonin as a sleep aid), you will soon have key take-home points and key information from dozens and dozens of resources well organized and at your fingertips. As a bonus, the tactile learning you do while making the table reinforces your learning and knowledge acquisition about your topic.

CONCLUSION

In this chapter, you have seen that every piece of scholarly writing begins with a question, and these questions often come from topics that you are passionate about or problems you want to solve. You have seen that becoming knowledgeable about a topic requires you go beyond your personal experiences and opinions to seek out a bigger picture. Reviewing published literature on a topic allows you to learn about where the state of the science is on the topic. What have people already done? What has worked or not worked to solve a problem? Most importantly, what still needs to be done? What can you add to the knowledge base on the topic? Remember that you do not have to collect every piece of information that has ever been published on a topic to start writing.

I know what it is like to be in "analysis paralysis," where it seems like there is so much information that there is nothing left for you to add to the discussion. A body of knowledge is built by the efforts of many and includes people's opinions, research study results, arguments, rebuttals to arguments, and a constant presentation of new ideas (or new ways of approaching old ideas). Think about how crucial the nurse's role is in the healthcare process, and know that what you have to say *is important*. I look forward to reading your work!

REFERENCES

Balfour, L., Kowal, J., Silverman, A., Tasca, G. A., Angel, J. B., Macpherson, P. A., . . . Cameron, D. W. (2006). A randomized controlled psycho-education intervention trial: Improving psychological readiness for successful HIV medication adherence and reducing depression before initiating HAART. *AIDS Care, 18*(7), 830–838. doi:10.1080/09540120500466820

Centers for Disease Control and Prevention. (2017). *HIV: basic statistics.* Retrieved from https://www.cdc.gov/hiv/basics/statistics.html

De Santis, J., & Barroso, S. (2011). Living in silence: A grounded theory study of vulnerability in the context of HIV infection. *Issues in Mental Health Nursing, 32*(6), 345–354. doi:10.3109/01612840.2010.550018

Garrard, J. (2016). *Health sciences literature review made easy.* Burlington, MA: Jones & Bartlett Publishers.

Gazza, E. A., Shellenbarger, T., & Hunker, D. F. (2013). Developing as a scholarly writer: The experience of students enrolled in a PhD in nursing program in the United States. *Nurse Education Today, 33*(3), 268–274. doi:10.1016/j.nedt.2012.04.019

Melnyk, B. M., & Morrison-Beedy, D. (2012). *Intervention research: Designing, conducting, analyzing, and funding.* New York, NY: Springer Publishing.

U.S. Department of Health and Human Services [DHHS]. (2017). *Guidelines for the use of antiretroviral agents in HIV-1-infected adults and adolescents.* Retrieved from https://aidsinfo.nih.gov/guidelines/html/1/adult-and-adolescent-treatment-guidelines/0/

World Health Organization [WHO]. (2017). *HIV/AIDS data and statistics.* Geneva, Switzerland: World Health Organization. Retrieved from http://www.who.int/hiv/data/en/

APPENDIX 3.1 RUNNING DOCUMENT TEMPLATE

HIV Infection

Topic	Data	Source
Global statistics	36.7 million infections worldwide 1.8 million new infections in 2016 1 million deaths from AIDS in 2016	(World Health Organization, 2017)
National statistics	1.1 million infections nationally **39,513 new infections in 2015** 6,721 HIV-related deaths in 2015	(Centers for Disease Control and Prevention, 2017)
Characteristics of high- risk individuals	Unprotected sexual intercourse • Unprotected, receptive anal and vaginal intercourse = highest risk Mother living with HIV; untreated = higher risk for mother-to-child transmission Multiple partners Needle sharing/needle stick • Injection drug use • Healthcare profession Biting/spitting/splashing = negligible risk	(Centers for Disease Control and Prevention, 2017)
Treatment options for HIV	Antiretroviral therapy: Targets stages of HIV lifecycle Reverse transcriptase inhibitors (NRTI/NNRTI) Protease inhibitors: 　Entry inhibitors 　Integrase inhibitors 　Fusion inhibitors	**(United States Department of Health and Human Services, 2017)**
State of HIV care in the United States	85% of all infected individuals have been diagnosed; others do not know they are infected 62% receiving care 48% retained in care 49% virally suppressed	(Centers for Disease Control and Prevention, 2017)

In the left column, determine the information that you want to collect. In this example, up-to-date global and national statistics about HIV in 2017

Place the statistic, fact, figure, or other piece of information in the middle column. This information will likely be updated over time as you read and as more scientific literature is released. In many cases (such as our example), agencies will update their statistics annually. Always make sure you are getting the most up to date statistics before writing.

For each piece of information, make sure you are documenting where the information came from so you can easily insert citations and references as you write. Use reference manager programs to help you organize the literature and easily insert references into your documents.

APPENDIX 3.2 LITERATURE REVIEW TABLE

In my dissertation work, I aimed at understanding the process of care initiation by people living with HIV. I needed to do thoroughly explore both quantitative and qualitative studies to learn about HIV care initiation. I needed to get an idea of what has been done and where there was a need for more knowledge. Reviewing the literature helped me to narrow my focus until I had a completely articulated idea of what I wanted to study. The template following includes a couple of the studies I reviewed as an example of abstracting data from published articles.

Authors	Purpose	Sample/Methods	Results/Contribution to Your Project
(De Santis & Barroso, 2011)	To describe, using qualitative methodology, the process by which vulnerability occurs in the context of HIV infection	**HIV-positive adults** (**N = 15**) **Grounded Theory:** • **In-depth inter views**	**Theory:** *Living in Silence* **Confronting mortality and illness Struggling with change Encountering a lack of psychosocial support Experiencing Vulnerability** Theory provides strong evidence for this dissertation study. This theory explores the vulnerability concept in terms of diagnosis, treatment side effects, AIDS-defining illnesses and symptoms, etc.

Descriptions of the sample, sample size, and specific methods used are useful for helping you see opportunities for future research or to identify methodological limitations in research that has been done.

After reading the article, list important take-home points or themes.

It is very helpful to always add a statement about why the research contributes to your work, or what the study in the row is missing that your research will fill. This will help you build strong arguments in your writing.

(continued)

Authors	Purpose	Sample/Methods	Results/Contribution to Your Project
(Balfour et al., 2006)	To evaluate a novel psychosocial educational intervention intended to increase patients' medication preparedness and treatment adherence skills BEFORE the initiation of antiretroviral therapy.	HIV-positive patients not currently on HAART ($N = 63$) Randomized control trial evaluating the Supportive Therapy for Adherence to Antiretroviral Treatments (STAART) Four-session psycho-educational intervention including baseline and follow-up measures to the 75-minute educational intervention	**Results:** STAART → increased medication readiness and decreased depression scores ($p<0.05$) **Contribution**: Treatment rReadiness is of great importance in HIV patients. The study demonstrates that both mental health and educational factors (psychosocial factors) contribute to readiness, a crucial factor in long-term success in HIV therapy. Dissertation gets into further detail about this time frame in the HIV care continuum.

An Example Paragraph Built from the Running Document and Literature Review Table

To illustrate, I have created an introductory paragraph based on the running document and literature table examples I have placed in this chapter.

More than 1 million people in the United States are living with human immunodeficiency **virus** (HIV; Centers for Disease Control and Prevention [CDC], 2017). Despite the availability of effective **treatment** (U.S. Department of Health and Human Services [DHHS], 2017), less than half of all people living with HIV in the United States are achieving viral **suppression** (CDC, 2017). In addition to coping with changes to their physical health after diagnosis, people living with HIV may also contend with psychosocial **challenges** (e.g., lack of social support, vulnerability; De Santis & Barroso, 2011). There is an urgent need for interventions to optimize entry into the HIV care environment in order to help people living with HIV establish and maintain viral **suppression**. The purpose of this study is to end the example paragraph because the reader likely gets the picture by now.

National Statistics from Running Document (hooks the reader).

Treatment statistics from Running Document.

De Santis and Barroso's article from Literature Table.

Statement of need to give the overall impact of the statistics and background information provided.

DHHS guidelines on antiretroviral therapy online article taken from Running Document.

CHAPTER 4

EVERYTHING BEGINS AND ENDS WITH AN OUTLINE

Robert Topp

PERSONAL STORY

A few years ago, I was invited as a member of the *Western Journal of Nursing Research* Editorial Board to contribute to a manuscript titled "Time Management Strategies for Research Productivity" (Chase et al., 2013). The editor asked me to develop a two- to three-page essay describing time management strategies that have contributed to my research success. I thought this was going to be the easiest publication I have ever authored for several reasons. First, I was sure I could "knock out" in about an hour two to three pages of advice based on personal experience that didn't require any literature review or background work. Second, I had developed an extensive repertoire of time management strategies on this topic. Third, many students and colleagues have complimented the time management strategies I provided to them because those strategies seemed to make them more productive. Fourth, I had 3 hours of unscheduled time on Friday afternoon to compose my contribution. Finally, if I finished the first draft of this manuscript within 3 hours I would reward myself by going to the beach to see the finals of the dog surfing contest. I thought I had all of the essential ingredients for a productive day: uninterrupted time to work, clear content to write about that didn't require any preparation in reviewing the literature, and motivation in the form of a really cool reward for my effort. When Friday afternoon arrived, I jumped right into writing the manuscript content. I did not want to waste time outlining information I knew and, therefore, risk missing the human and canine tandem surf competition. I began by writing about time management strategies, and how these strategies worked under different circumstances with different people and when completing different tasks. I wrote about which components of writing a data-based manuscript took more time, the importance of having a reviewer critique your work, and the challenges of writing in groups versus alone. After I found myself advising the reader about punctuation and grammar, I decided that writing this manuscript was much harder than I originally had thought. The document I had produced at this point read like a bunch of random disconnected thoughts and the content had seriously drifted from the original topic: describing time management strategies that contributed to my research success. Why was this document not coming together? Then it dawned on me. I failed to take time to generate an outline of this manuscript and without an outline I did not have a clear guide about what I wanted to say or to keep me from drifting into irrelevant topics. I "reloaded" using a yellow legal pad and wrote down the three main topics I wanted to cover in this manuscript. I added some content in the form of bullet points that I wanted to cover within each of these topics. I rearranged the topics and content into a logical order and then I began composing a new manuscript. After spending 20 minutes drafting this outline, I found the manuscript much easier to write. I focused on the three topics in the outline and resisted the temptation to drift into interesting but irrelevant topics. I kept reminding myself that if the topic was not in my outline, then I did not include it in my manuscript. Most importantly, I finished the first draft of the manuscript just in time to see the finals of the dog surfing competition.

INTRODUCTION

Once again, I learned the hard way the valuable lesson of how developing an outline prior to starting to write a scholarly manuscript makes writing the actual manuscript much easier. As the story indicated, trying to write even a section of a manuscript about a topic, even a familiar one, was difficult without first creating an outline as a guide in developing the content and structure. To keep you from repeating my mistake, I developed this chapter. The purpose of this chapter is to describe how to develop and use an outline when writing a scholarly manuscript. The first section of this chapter explains the disadvantages and advantages of creating an outline before beginning to write a scholarly manuscript. Next, I discuss how first developing a clear purpose and a logical argument will guide formation of your outline and eventually your manuscript. With a purpose and logical argument, I then demonstrate the process of developing an outline. Finally, based on an outline, I provide an example of composing an introduction for a scholarly manuscript. The appendices to this chapter include a template for creating an outline for a data-based manuscript (Appendix 4.1), a research proposal (Appendix 4.2), and a non–data-based manuscript (Appendix 4.3).

OUTLINES

(Dis)advantages of an Outline

> **WRITING TIP**
> Developing an outline will keep you from being "distracted by shiny objects" that aren't relevant to the new knowledge you want to communicate in your manuscript. "Shiny objects" are REALLY interesting topics you find attention-grabbing but do not belong in your manuscript.

There are many advantages to developing an outline before you begin writing a scholarly manuscript. In contrast to these advantages, I frequently hear many "reasons" from emerging scholars for not developing an outline prior to beginning to write a scholarly manuscript. Some of the more creative explanations are listed in Box 4.1. I will not dignify any of the reasons in Box 4.1 for not developing an outline with a response since I am sure that if you invest time in developing an outline prior to beginning a scholarly manuscript, you *will* realize a number of positive outcomes. First, and probably most importantly, when you develop an outline you will develop a logical presentation of your ideas that will clearly support the new knowledge you will reveal in the manuscript. Scientific writing requires special attention to order and organization, which is what an outline provides prior to composing large sections of the manuscript. Second, contrary to reason number one in Box 4.1, once you develop an outline you may be able to copy sections of the outline into the first draft of your manuscript. Commonly, the purpose statement you develop in your outline will be the same purpose statement you include in your manuscript. Within your outline you may also develop introductory or transition sentences for specific sections that you can also use in your manuscript. Developing an outline commonly includes components you write once but can use twice: once in the outline and again in the manuscript. The third reason to develop an outline is that, prior to writing entire sections, it allows you to critically analyze the logical progression of your ideas and experiment with various ordering of the content. The ability to change the ordering of the content before you write the content allows you to find the best order and a fluid logical sequence for the knowledge you are presenting. Ordering the sequence of your manuscript first allows you to compose clear transitions and linkages between the content areas instead of attempting to compose the content, logically order the content, and provide transitions between the content areas simultaneously. Fourth, developing an outline saves time when writing the manuscript. The outline clearly plans the content of the manuscript. Taking time to create an outline allows you to understand and see the content you will write about and perhaps more importantly, excludes content you will not write about. When teaching colleagues how to write from an outline, I tell them "if the content is not written on the outline then you do not include the content in the manuscript." An outline can also be used to budget the space of the final manuscript. For example, if you have a 10-page limit to your manuscript you may anticipate half a page each for the introduction (beginning) and conclusion (end), which leaves you nine pages for the content (middle). Depending on the number of sections and the emphasis you wish to place on each of the sections, you can roughly budget a page limit to each of the manuscript sections. Using this 10-page limit example, if you are proposing three sections with similar emphasis in your manuscript, your outline indicates allocating approximately three pages for each section. The advantages of an outline far outweigh the disadvantages since creating an outline will help you develop and logically organize the content and guide you in what to include and *not* include in your manuscript.

BOX 4.1: REASONS* FOR NOT DEVELOPING AN OUTLINE

1. Developing an outline is like writing the same thing twice.

2. I do not need an outline if I know what I want to write.

3. Following an outline constrains my creative process.

4. If I adhere to an outline, I cannot change the direction of the manuscript as I learn more about the content.

5. For a manuscript assigned for an academic class, the instructor provides the outline in the form of the instructions for the assignment.

6. If I have given a presentation on the topic, such as a poster or a lecture, I do not need to develop an outline for a manuscript based upon the presentation.

7. I do not want to be the same as everyone else – creating an outline (e.g., purpose statement, etc.) puts me in a box.

8. I do not want to miss the surfing dog competition (or other equally awesome event).

*None of these reasons for not developing an outline outweigh the advantages to developing an outline prior to writing a scholarly manuscript (as tempting as surfing dogs may be).

Before Developing an Outline

The first step in developing an outline for a scholarly manuscript is to identify the purpose of the manuscript that clearly states the new knowledge you wish to communicate. Sometimes identifying the purpose is plainly prescribed by the instructions for a course assignment or when

WRITING TIP

Using the rule of three is a common way you learned and remember information:

- Stop, look, and listen.
- "Life, liberty, and the pursuit of happiness."
- "Government of the people, by the people, for the people"
- Truth, justice, and the American way.
- Duty - honor - country.
- Bacon, lettuce, and tomato
- Larry, Curley, and Moe

writing a data-based manuscript that addresses the purpose of a research project. Other times the purpose of a scholarly manuscript must be distilled from an idea of new knowledge the author wishes to communicate. This distillation may require the author to refine the idea for the new knowledge after reviewing what knowledge currently exists in the area. The purpose clearly describes the new knowledge the reader realizes from reading the scholarly manuscript. The remaining sections of the manuscript are all directed at achieving the stated purpose of the manuscript. Once you have written the purpose of your scholarly manuscript, all the sections of the manuscript must provide a clear, logical progression of content to achieve the purpose. Any content in your manuscript that does not contribute to the purpose will confuse the reader by distracting them from the new knowledge you wish to communicate. When developing the logical progression of your content to achieve the purpose of your manuscript, try to follow the "Rule of Three" (Clark, 2015). The Rule of Three is a principle of writing that indicates content presented in groupings of three are more effective at communicating the message and engaging the reader. The ancient Romans coined the term "omne trium perfectum," which means everything in three is perfect. Presenting content in groupings of three is pervasive in literature. For example, "The Three Little Pigs" (Foreman, 1952), "The Three Musketeers" (Dumas, 1994), "The Oedipus Trilogy" (Spender & Sophocles, 1985), or the three lines in a Haiku. Three is also the basic story telling structure of writing a play or a screenplay (Field, 2007). The three-part structure for telling a story is the structure readers are most familiar with reading and thus, readers are comfortable with and even expect a story in three parts: the beginning, the middle, and the end. When developing an outline for a scholarly manuscript, write the purpose and then attempt to support the purpose with three clear, logically connected points, all of which are directed at achieving the purpose. For example, imagine you wish to compose a scholarly manuscript with the following purpose.

Notice how the exact terms stated in the purpose are used when describing the three major content areas that will achieve the purpose

The **purpose** of this manuscript is to describe how a nurse can employ a model of communication as the framework for developing a YouTube video to discuss palliative care with a caregiver of a dementia patient.

Notice how the first section will develop definitions for all of the terms mentioned in the purpose so the author and reader share a common definition of these terms

The next step is to identify and logically order the three major content areas that will contribute to achieving the purpose:

1. **Define terms** (*palliative care, caregiver of dementia patients, nurse, YouTube video*).

> This model of communication is existing knowledge upon which the author will build new knowledge.

2. *Explain the components of a **model** of communication (information, transmitter, channel, receiver).*

3. ***Construct a framework*** *using the model to discuss palliative care with caregivers of dementia patients. (Palliative care = information; nurse = transmitter; YouTube video = channel; caregiver = receiver.)*

> This final section is the new knowledge that is being communicated in the manuscript and combines the terms with the components of the model.

As mentioned throughout this text, a scholarly manuscript communicates new knowledge that is based upon existing knowledge, with consistent language in a format specific to the discipline (Gazza, Shellenbarger, & Hunker, 2013). An outline provides the framework upon which a scholarly manuscript is built. In other words, an outline summarizes all the major points to be included in the manuscript *and* the logical order in which the points will be presented. The starting point of a scholarly manuscript is to identify the new knowledge that will be disclosed in the manuscript. This new knowledge is commonly expressed as the purpose and tells the reader what new knowledge will be revealed in the manuscript. Thus, the first step in developing an outline is to write down the purpose of the manuscript. By doing so, you begin to refine and narrow the focus and content of your manuscript. Writing down the purpose instead of "knowing" or having the purpose "in mind" allows you constantly return to and remind yourself of the new knowledge you want to communicate and minimizes the possibility that the purpose of your manuscript will drift to other topics.

WRITING TIP

Now you know why we made you take logic and rhetoric as required courses in college. It wasn't all about if a tree falls in the forest with no one there to hear it. . . .The principles of developing an argument taught in these courses are critical when developing a scholarly manuscript.

After you develop the preliminary purpose of your manuscript, you will need to develop a logical argument that supports the validity or soundness of the purpose or new knowledge. The new knowledge you present in your manuscript can be thought of as the conclusion of an argument and the sections supporting the new knowledge can be considered the supporting premises to an argument's conclusion. There are two broad types of logical arguments that can be applied to composing a scholarly manuscript: deductive and inductive. A deductive argument states that the validity of a conclusion is a logical consequence of the premises. If the premises of a deductive argument are true, then it simply is not possible for the conclusion to be false. In other words, within a deductive argument, the validity of the conclusion is dependent upon the validity of the premises. In a deductive argument if the premises are not true, then the conclusion will not be valid. For example, a valid deductive argument may be, "Lauren is an author. All authors work hard. Therefore, Lauren works hard." Notice that the validity of the conclusion, Lauren works hard, is dependent on the validity of the two preceding premises.

The other type of logical argument is an inductive argument. This type of argument states that the truth of the conclusion is supported to some degree by the probability of the premises. In an inductive argument, if the premises are likely true, it is improbable that the conclusion would be false. Thus, the validity of the conclusion in an inductive argument is built upon the probably that the premises are valid. An example of an inductive argument is, "Most authors work hard. Lauren is an author. Therefore, Lauren probably works hard."

Now that you have endured a refresher course in structuring logical arguments, I want to explain how a logical argument will assist you in building your outline. Premises of an argument are developed to logically support the conclusion of an argument. The validity or truth of the conclusion is based on the validity or truth of the premises. Similarly, the new knowledge you disclose in your manuscript, stated in the purpose, must also be supported by evidence or pre-existing knowledge. The new knowledge you disclose is only as valid as the evidence supporting the new knowledge. This evidence can be in the form of results of empirical studies, expert opinions, or logically derived from proposed theoretical relationships among constructs. The first level of your outline includes the major sections that logically support the overall purpose or new knowledge you wish disclose in your manuscript. Each of these major sections may be divided into smaller components termed "topics," which may, in turn, be divided and supported by "subtopics," which may be again partitioned and supported by "sub-subtopics," all of which provide evidence for the next higher level in the hierarchy of the outline. For example, you wish to develop a manuscript that describe elements of an effective program that decreases healthcare acquired infections (HCAIs) in an acute care hospital. The new knowledge you wish to communicate in this manuscript is to describe an effective program that decreases HCAI in an acute care hospital that includes both changes in nursing practice and changes in the organization's policies. Thus, the purpose of this manuscript must be to discuss an effective program that decreases HCAI in an acute care hospital that includes both changes in nursing practice and changes in the organization's policies. Box 4.2 presents an inductive argument that provides the framework for this manuscript.

Constructing an Outline

Translating this logical argument into a manuscript outline involves organizing the structure of the outline into three broad areas: the beginning (introduction), the middle (content), and the end (conclusion). The introduction commonly includes three components and the outline lists each of these components. First, the introduction includes the "hook" or

BOX 4.2: AN INDUCTIVE ARGUMENT

Notice how this argument employs the "rule of three." The three premises build upon each other and support the conclusion

P1: Healthcare acquired infections (HCAIs) are a significant problem in acute care hospitals.

P2: Changes in nursing practice are associated with decreases in HCAIs.

P3: Changes in organizational policy are associated with decreases in HCAIs.

C: Therefore, elements of an effective program that decreases the significant problem of HCAIs in an acute care hospital can include both changes in nursing practice and changes in the organization's policies.

the unresolved problem that the new knowledge revealed in the manuscript will attempt to address. Second, the purpose of the manuscript, or a statement of the new knowledge that the manuscript will reveal, is mentioned in the introduction. This purpose explains how the manuscript will address the unresolved problem mentioned in the hook. Finally, the introduction includes an explanation of the structure and content of the structure of the manuscript by which the purpose will be achieved. This final section of an introduction provides a roadmap to the reader regarding the order and content of the upcoming sections of the manuscript. These sections need to be organized logically and consistently based upon the premises and conclusion of the argument. For example, it confuses the reader if you present the conclusion or new knowledge prior to stating the premises, supporting evidence, or previously established knowledge. As well, it is odd to present premises or supporting evidence for new knowledge without first stating the problem the new knowledge will address. Thus, this final section of the introduction not only explains the content to be covered in the manuscript, but also the structure or order in which the content will be presented. Exhibit 4.1 presents an outline of a manuscript based upon the inductive argument assembled in Box 4.2.

From Outline to Introduction

As Box 4.2 and Exhibit 4.1 demonstrate, developing an outline progresses from stating the purpose or new knowledge to be presented in the manuscript followed by developing a logical argument that supports the purpose and then expanding and logically ordering the content of the logical argument into an outline. The outline presented in Exhibit 4.1 includes topics, subtopics, and sub-subtopics. These components are presented as bullets, phrases, or sentences. Bullets or phrases provide the author with a topical area or point to develop that supports the next

EXHIBIT 4.1: MANUSCRIPT OUTLINE

An effective introduction includes three components:

1. A "hook" or problem
2. A purpose or new knowledge to be disclosed
3. A description of the structure of the manuscript and the content of the structure

1. **Introduction (Beginning)**

   a. **Hook: The prevalence of healthcare acquired infections (HCAIs) among hospitalized inpatients in developed countries including the United States is estimated to be between 5% and 12% (Allegranzi, Nejad, & Pittet, 2017).** HCAIs kill or make sick a lot of patients. HCAIs cost the hospital, third party providers, and patients money.

   First sentence of the manuscript?

   The hook states a problem that the manuscript will address and explains to the reader some undesirable phenomena or problem in need of being fixed.

   b. **The purpose of this manuscript is to describe an effective program that decreases HCAIs in an acute care hospital that includes both changes in nursing practice and changes in the organization's policies.**

   Notice how the purpose of the manuscript is similar to the conclusion of the inductive argument

   c. Explain the structure and content of the structure of the manuscript

      i. Problem of HCAIs

      ii. Nursing practice and HCAIs

      iii. Organizational policies and HCAIs

      iv. Present a new program to decrease HCAIs including changes in nursing practice and organizational policies

   This section of the manuscript is consistent with the first premise in the argument. This section will provide evidence that supports the validity of the premise that HCAI are a problem in acute care hospitals.

2. **Content (Middle)**

   a. **The problem of HCAIs in acute care hospitals**

      i. Define an HCAIs

      ii. **Scope of the problem**

   This topic discussing the scope of HACIs supports the section that HCAIs are a problem

         □ **How many HCAIs per year prevalence and incidence**

   This subtopic including incidence and prevalence of HCAIs supports the topic of the scope of HCAI in hospitals

      iii. **Significance of the problem**

         □ Cost of HCAIs to the patient, hospital, insurance company and society

   The significance of the problem explains the impact of the problem in terms of cost, morbidity and mortality &/or declines in quality of life

         □ Impact of HCAIs on the patient's quality of life in the hospital and beyond

         □ Rate of death or lasting disability from HCAIs

   b. The impact of nursing practice on HCAIs in an acute care hospital

(continued)

EXHIBIT 4.1: MANUSCRIPT OUTLINE*(continued)*

    i. Explain how nursing practice contributes to HCAIs

        ☐ Contact with many patients

        ☐ Practices that contribute to HCAIs

    ii. Changes in nursing practice decrease HCAIs

        ☐ Individual nursing practice

        a. **Regular hand washing, use of personal protective supplies**

        ☐ Unit nursing practice

        b. Assigning nurses to adjacent rooms, provide access to personal protection supplies

Notice how sub-subtopics provide evidence for the next higher level in the hierarchy of the outline. Hand washing is a component of personal nursing practice which in turn supports changes in nursing practice that finally provides evidence to support the impact of nursing practice on HCAI in an acute care hospital

  c. The impact of organizational policy on HCAIs in an acute care hospital

    i. Explain how organization policies contribute to HCAIs

        ☐ Policies on nursing staffing ratios

        ☐ Policies on nursing self-governance to address HCAIs

    ii. Review the literature for interventions on how a change in organizational policies effect HCAIs

        ☐ Studies describing relationships between organizational policies and HCAIs

        ☐ Interventional studies examining the effect of a change in organizational policies on HCAIs

This is the section of the manuscript that addresses the purpose of the manuscript by presenting the new knowledge

This sentence could be used as the first sentence introducing this section in the first draft of the manuscript.

    iii. **Based on the current evidence, an effective program that decreases HCAIs in an acute care hospital includes two broad components:**

        ☐ Changes in nursing practice

        ☐ Changes in the organization's policies

Remind the reader of the problem the manuscript is attempting to address

3. **Conclusion (End)**

  a. **HCAIs are a big problem**

  b. **An effective program that decreases HCAIs in an acute care hospital includes changes in nursing practice and organizational policies**

Reiterate in the conclusion how the manuscript achieved the purpose

higher level in the outline hierarchy. A sentence in an outline may be based upon some pre-existing knowledge, evidence from the literature, or a logical argument developed as the framework of the manuscript. The more pre-existing knowledge you are familiar with, the more sentences you will probably be able to include in your outline—sentences that you can transfer into the first draft of your manuscript. The outline provides a framework for your manuscript and can be translated easily into the introduction of the manuscript. Recall that the introduction section of a manuscript includes the hook or a statement of the scope and significance of the problem. The hook is followed by the purpose of the manuscript or the new knowledge that will be communicated. Finally, the introduction explains the structure and content of the structure of the manuscript by which the purpose will be achieved. Exhibit 4.2 is an introduction based upon the outline in Exhibit 4.1. Since this outline was fairly detailed, much of the content of the introduction is directly transferred from this outline into the introduction of the manuscript. The outline clearly articulated the content and the order of the content so composing the introduction easily followed this content and order.

EXHIBIT 4.2: INTRODUCTION BASED UPON THE OUTLINE

The scope of the problem.

The prevalence of health care acquired infections (HCAIs) among hospitalized inpatients in developed countries including the United States is estimated to be between 5% and 12% (Allegranzi et al., 2017). Applying two different Consumer Price Index (CPI) adjustments to account for the rate of inflation in hospital resource prices, the overall annual direct medical costs of HCAIs to U.S. hospitals ranges from $28.4 to $33.8 billion (Scott, 2009). Umscheid et al. (2011) have suggested that up to 75% of HCAIs are preventable. Other researchers have reported changes in nursing practice (McNeill, 2017) or changes in organizational policies (Zingg et al., 2015) are effective strategies

Overtly stated purpose of the manuscript or new knowledge to be presented.

to prevent HCAIs. **The purpose** of this manuscript is to describe an effective program that decreases HCAIs in an acute care hospital that includes both changes in nursing practice and changes in the organization's policies. **This manuscript will achieve this purpose by**

The explanation of the structure and content of the structure of the manuscript by which the purpose will be achieved.

first describing the scope and significance of HCAIs. This section will be followed by describing how changes in nursing practice at the individual and unit practice level can reduce HCAIs in acute care hospitals. The third section of this manuscript will present how HCAIs are affected by changes in organizational policies. Following these three sections, the final portion of the manuscript will present a new program to decrease HCAIs including changes in nursing practice and organizational policies.

CONCLUSION

After reading this chapter, I hope you are starting to realize that scientific writing aims to communicate new knowledge through a purposeful, consistent, structured approach. There are many advantages that outweigh the few weak disadvantages to developing an outline prior to beginning to write a scholarly manuscript. Before developing an outline, you need to identify the purpose or new knowledge you wish to communicate and then develop a logical argument to support the purpose. In this chapter, I demonstrated how to take a purpose statement and a logical argument and develop an outline for a scholarly manuscript. This outline employed the literary Rule of Three, which facilitates the communication and comprehension of the new knowledge. Finally, I developed an introductory paragraph for a scholarly manuscript based upon the outline. Throughout this chapter, I attempted to demonstrate how the purpose statement is supported by the logical argument, how the logical argument provides the basis for major sections in the outline, how the outline drives the content of the introduction of the manuscript, and how the introduction of the manuscript informs the reader of the content of the entire scholarly manuscript.

REFERENCES

Allegranzi, B., Nejad, S. B., & Pittet, D. (2017). The burden of healthcare-associated infection. *Hand hygiene: A handbook for medical professionals* (pp. 1–7). Hoboken, NJ: John Wiley & Sons.

Chase, J. A., Topp, R., Smith, C. E., Cohen, M. Z., Fahrenwald, N., Zerwic, J. J., . . . Conn, V. S. (2013). Time management strategies for research productivity. *Western Journal of Nursing Research, 35*(2), 155–176. doi:10.1177/0193945912451163

Clark, B. (2015). *How to use the "Rule of Three" to create engaging content.* Retrieved from https://www.copyblogger.com/rule-of-three

Dumas, A. (1994). *The three musketeers.* London, UK: Macmillan.

Field, S. (2007). *Screenplay: The foundations of screenwriting.* New York, NY: Delta.

Foreman, G. F. (1952). *Three little pigs.* Rockville Centre, NY: Belwin.

Gazza, E. A., Shellenbarger, T., & Hunker, D. F. (2013). Developing as a scholarly writer: The experience of students enrolled in a PhD in nursing program in the United States. *Nurse Education Today, 33*(3), 268–274. doi:10.1016/j.nedt.2012.04.019

McNeill, L. (2017). Back to basics: How evidence-based nursing practice can prevent catheter-associated urinary tract infections. *Urologic Nursing, 37*(4), 204–206. doi:10.7257/1053- 816X.2017.37.4.204

Scott, R. D. (2009). *The direct medical costs of healthcare-associated infections in U.S. hospitals and the benefits of prevention.* Retrieved from https://www.cdc.gov/hai/pdfs/hai/scott_costpaper.pdf

Spender, S., & Sophocles. (1985). *Oedipus trilogy: King oedipus, oedipus at colonos, antigone.* New York, NY: Random House.

Umscheid, C. A., Mitchell, M. D., Doshi, J. A., Agarwal, R., Williams, K., & Brennan, P. J. (2011). Estimating the proportion of healthcare-associated infections that are reasonably preventable and the related mortality and costs. *Infection Control & Hospital Epidemiology, 32*(2), 101–114. doi:10.1086/657912

Zingg, W., Holmes, A., Dettenkofer, M., Goetting, T., Secci, F., Clack, L., . . . Pittet, D. (2015). Hospital organisation, management, and structure for prevention of health-care-associated infection: A systematic review and expert consensus. *The Lancet Infectious Diseases, 15*(2), 212–224. doi:10.1016/S1473-3099(14)70854-0

APPENDIX 4.1 OUTLINE TEMPLATE FOR DATA-BASED MANUSCRIPTS

Background

- Describe the scope and significance of an unresolved problem
- Describe previous evidence from the literature that attempted to address this problem
- Based on this previous evidence provide a logical argument for conducting the study to be presented in the manuscript.

The purpose of a data - based manuscript includes three components:

1. The variables being studied
2. How the variables are being studied (describe, relationships, cause and effect)
3. The population being studied

Purpose

The purpose of this study is to [describe variables] or [determine the relationships between variables] or [determine the effect of (independent variable on dependent variables)] among [population]

Hypotheses/Research Questions/Aims/Objectives

Methodology

- Design
- Sample and setting
- Intervention
- Data collection

- Protocol
- Data management and analysis plan

Results

- Descriptive analysis of the sample
- Analysis that addresses the Hypotheses/Research Questions/Aims/Objectives
- Tables/figures/graphs presenting the results of the analysis

Conclusion/Discussion

- How do the results of the data analysis support/refute the hypotheses/answer the research questions/achieve the aims of objectives?
- How do the results address the purpose or the unresolved problem stated in the background?
- Are the findings consistent with previous evidence from the literature supporting the need for the current study?
- How can the results be used to support future research, changes in clinical practice and/or theoretical relationships between the variables being studied?

APPENDIX 4.2 OUTLINE TEMPLATE FOR RESEARCH PROPOSALS

Problem Statement:

- Present the problem you are addressing with this study in term of cost ($), health implications including morbidity and mortality (M&M) or declines in quality of life (QOL)
- Discuss this problem in terms of the scope—how many affected and the significance—the degree to which the problem affects cost, morbidity and mortality, and quality of life
- Provide definitions of the variables you will be studying and the population you will be studying **AND use only these labels of the variables and the population consistently throughout the proposal**
- This section should leave the reader thinking "someone needs to study this problem" and thus justify your purpose

Background: Provides a more complete exploration of the problem in order to justify your purpose. Commonly follows the outline you use in your problem statement section:

- Define the problem in the population
- Discuss what has been done about this problem and why this has or has not worked may involve similar populations or similar (but not exactly your) interventions
- Discuss why the problem persists (gaps)
- Discuss the potential of your study to address the problem, which justifies the need for your study!

Purpose: ALWAYS BEGINS WITH THESE SIX WORDS "The purpose of this study is to. . .." followed by one of these three phrases

1. Describe X and Y [this is a descriptive study in which you intend to describe some phenomenon that has yet to be described or measured]
2. Determine the relationships between X and Y [this is a correlational study in which you are determining how variables are associated or how one variable is predicated from other variables]
3. The effect of X on Y [this is an intervention study in which you are measuring the effect of X (independent variable(s) or the intervention) on Y (the dependent or outcome variables)]

The purpose statement also includes the population of interest by saying *among [Z group of individuals].*

When restating the purpose always cut and paste the same purpose sentence throughout your proposal.

Provide a linking sentence from the purpose to the research questions (RQ)/research hypotheses (RH); e.g., this purpose will be achieved by addressing the following hypotheses or answering the following research questions.

Research Questions:

- RQ1: Are questions and are appropriate for descriptive and some correlational studies when evidence is lacking and it is necessary to make an educated guess about describing the variables or predicting how the variables go together [these question statements include the population of interest and end in a "?"]

Research Hypotheses

- RH1: Hypotheses are educated guesses based upon previous evidence about how variables go together and are expressed in declarative statements ending in a "."

Methods

- Design: Provides an overall description of who does what, when, how, where, and why in order to achieve the purpose.

The proposed study is a ____ design in which subjects will _____ and be measured _____.

Sample: Describes the characteristics of the group you will study (inclusion and exclusion criteria); describes how you will recruit this group; and how you decided on the size of the sample you are studying.

Protocol or Intervention: (May not have this section depending on study design) Describes how subjects progress through the protocol starting with providing consent, when data collection takes place, and the how the intervention (if being studied) is applied. This section should be so clear that after reading it anyone could conduct the study.

Outcome Measures: Describes how each variable you mention in the purpose or RQ/RHs will be measured. This description may include psychometric properties of the data collection procedure (e.g. validity and reliability) as well as qualifications of the persons collecting the data.

Analysis: Describes how data will be transferred from the data collection protocol to a spread sheet; describes preliminary analysis to support inferential statistics. Describes specific statistics to be conducted to address each RQ and RH.

Time Line

Describes project milestones and when they will be completed:

- Final proposal approval
- Institutional review board approval
- Begin study protocol
- Complete study protocol
- Complete analysis and preliminary report
- Submission for conference presentation
- Submission of manuscript for publication

Budget

Personnel (people who need to be paid because the study couldn't be done without them)

Equipment (things you can keep using after the study is over; e.g., computers)

Supplies (things you throw away but are essential to completing the study; e.g., blood tubes)

Other

- Subject incentives
- Consultation costs
- Food

- Other goods or services you need to purchase
- Costs associated with publishing or presenting the results

Travel

- Subjects traveling to you
- You traveling to subjects
- You and/or your team traveling to present

APPENDIX 4.3 OUTLINE TEMPLATE FOR A NON–DATA-BASED MANUSCRIPT

Outline template for a non–data-based manuscript

1. **Introduction (Beginning)**

   An effective introduction includes three components:

   1. A "hook" or problem.
   2. A purpose or new knowledge to be disclosed.
   3. A description of the structure of the manuscript and the content of the structure.

   - Hook including the significance and scope of the problem the new knowledge will address
   - The purpose of this manuscript is to_____
   - Explain the structure and content of the manuscript directed at achieving the purpose of the manuscript
     - i.   Section 1
     - ii.   Section 2
     - iii. Section . . .
     - iv.   Section that includes new knowledge

2. **Content (Middle)**

   Section 1

   Topics

   Subtopics

   Section 2

   Topics

   Subtopics

   Section . . .

   Topics . . .

   Subtopics. . .

   Section that includes the new knowledge

   Combining sections 1- . . . to present new knowledge

   Describe how the new knowledge addresses the problem in the hook

Describe implications for the new knowledge for clinical practice, future research and/or theory development

3. **Conclusion (End)**

Restate the hook or the problem

Summarize the structure and content of the structure

Summarize how the new knowledge addresses the problem

CHAPTER 5

TITLE AND ABSTRACT: IT'S THE SMALL STUFF THAT MATTERS

Robert Topp

PERSONAL STORY

I just finished writing what I was confident in saying was a well-written abstract for the first research project I conducted independently. I was very proud of this piece of new knowledge I was contributing to the world and I finished it 6 hours before the deadline set by the conference organizers. Before submitting my abstract, I ran a word count on the document and discovered my abstract was 483 words or 183 words over the 300-word limit stated in the instructions. No problem. I had 6 hours to sharpen my abstract so I started deleting words, shortening sentences, and clarifying the text. After this first rewrite to shorten the length of the document I ran the word count again—I had managed to only get it down to 456 words! I realized that sharpening and deleting were not going to get me to my goal of 300 words. I had not yet realized that I needed to delete one third of the current content of my abstract. With a moderate amount of discomfort, I started to delete entire sentences. No more mention of previous studies. No more next steps in the research trajectory. No more theoretical implications of the findings. My abstract was now down to 402 words with 4 hours to go until the deadline and I still had to cut 25% of the words in the document. It was time for drastic "scorched-earth" tough decisions about what was essential to be in my abstract. With great pain, I deleted the demographic description of my sample, the secondary findings, and the three sentence implications for practice.

Notice how I started to divorce myself from ownership of this abstract.

This "deflated balloon" abstract now contained 330 words. I could not find anything to cut without diluting the scientific merit of the work or make my abstract sound like it was written for a first grade student's reading primer. I started to think that this study could not be contained in 300 words and that the conference organizers were using this 300-word limit as a way of squelching important science. What to do? I now had 2 hours before the deadline and I started to wonder if anyone would notice if I deleted every 10th word. I considered developing even more arcane abbreviations (e.g., least significant difference or LSD). Getting this abstract to 300 words was taking me longer to produce than writing the first draft of the abstract. I finally asked a colleague for help and as a result of her "cold, impersonal, ruthless, editing," I submitted a 298-word abstract 15 minutes before the deadline. This story demonstrates the challenges everyone experiences in developing an abstract that clearly and succinctly communicates the new knowledge contained in the scholarly manuscript within a limited word count. This chapter is designed to help you write an abstract that balances these two **criteria.**

To give you a frame of reference: This not-so-succinct story was 468 words, almost the same length as my "well-written" abstract.

INTRODUCTION

My personal story shows what can sometimes be the hardest part of scholarly writing—to compose a document that clearly and succinctly communicates the new knowledge. This chapter begins by debunking a few myths about what must be included in a scholarly manuscript. Believing these myths sometimes paralyzes young scholars into not even beginning to write. I then discuss the content of the title of a scholarly manuscript and the importance of developing a title that is concise and describes the new knowledge revealed in the manuscript. Next, this chapter demonstrates how to develop an abstract for a scholarly manuscript. An abstract is an abbreviated, accurate representation of a document (Weil, 1970). An abstract is not a summary. A summary is a restatement of the substance of the work at the end of a section or at the end of the total work. An annotation is different than an abstract since an annotation contains one or two general statements about the substance of the work and serves as an extension of the title (Juhl & Norman, 1989). In the third section of this chapter, I present the formula and templates for composing data-based and non-data–based abstracts. Finally, I present an example of creating the first draft of a scholarly abstract and then revising this 600-word abstract to 300 words and ultimately, to a 150-word abstract. This example shows you how to clearly and succinctly communicate the new knowledge within an abstract.

MYTHS ABOUT SCHOLARLY MANUSCRIPTS

You are probably wondering why debunking myths about scholarly manuscripts is in this chapter about writing titles and abstracts. As I mentioned in the introduction, sometimes the hardest part of scholarly writing is composing a document that communicates new knowledge clearly and succinctly. Even before starting to write, some authors struggle to begin because they subscribe to widely held myths about what a scholarly manuscript must include to be published. The following are four widely held myths about what the content of a scholarly manuscript must include. Following each of these myths, I provide evidence in an attempt to debunk the myth, thereby reducing the barriers to clear and succinct writing.

Myth #1: Only Manuscripts With Broad Theoretical or Clinical Implications or Those That Significantly "Move" the Science Are Published

All myths are based in some measure on truth or reality. This myth is likely based on the fact that reading assignments in college commonly have broad implications and have formed the foundation for the scientific content that is being taught in the course. I remember reading a manuscript by Pender, Walker, Sechrist, and Frank-Stromborg (1990) titled "Predicting Health-Promoting Lifestyles in the Workplace." The manuscript concluded by indicating that internally controlled perceptions of health predicted if the individual would engage in health-promoting behaviors in the future. I imagined the new knowledge in this manuscript could have implications for every future clinical intervention designed to promote healthy behaviors. After reading this manuscript during my graduate studies I thought "How in the world will I ever be able to sit down and write a similar manuscript that has this kind of broad theoretical or clinical implications?" When examining the reference list of this manuscript and doing more literature search, I realized that these authors did not just sit down and write this manuscript. This manuscript was the result of years of preliminary studies resulting in numerous preliminary manuscripts that were narrowly focused with limited implications. These preliminary manuscripts described instrument development (Sechrist, Walker, & Pender, 1987), development of a conceptual framework (Pender & Pender, 1985), and preliminary studies with specific populations (Pender & Pender, 1985; Walker, Volkan, Sechrist, & Pender, 1988), all of which provided the basis for this study. Thus, very few published scholarly manuscripts have broad implications or have the potential to move the science. When you come across a manuscript that does have broad implications for theory or clinical application, that manuscript is usually born out of extensive preliminary work that results in manuscripts that may not have a tremendous impact on theories or clinical practice.

Myth #2: Only Manuscripts With Wide Appeal Will Be Published

This myth is one of my personal favorites because early in my academic career I tried to conduct research and write manuscripts on topics that I thought had a wide appeal. I pursued these topics because my mentors had advised me to study topics that I enjoyed or interested me. After talking with my family and friends about my research and sharing some of my early published manuscripts with them, I quickly realized that the topics I liked studying and writing about were really boring to almost everyone I knew. I vividly recall my father's expression after he tried reading one of my first scholarly abstracts; it was like his expression when I gave him a cracked, blue clay bowl I made in kindergarten, which still resides in a place of prominence in his home. His expression communicated that he was proud of my achievement but did not really know why. At the time, my disappointment that very few people shared my interest in what I was studying and writing about was buoyed by a single individual from Germany who contacted me and asked for a copy of one of the early manuscripts I had published. This single contact validated that at least one other person on the planet shared my scholarly interest. More recently, thanks to linking my manuscripts on various social media sites (e.g., LinkedIn, Research Gate, Facebook), I can see interest in my manuscripts sometimes swell to three downloads per month! Most scholarly manuscripts do not have a wide appeal because they are written with a narrow, specific focus and most people are not interested in that narrow and specific a topic.

Myth #3: Only Unique Manuscripts That Are Original Will Be Published

Scholarly manuscripts have to balance being too original, unique, or avant-garde with not offering any new knowledge. Scholarly content that is not firmly based on previously established knowledge is commonly considered unfounded or "too far out there." At the other end of the spectrum is scholarly content that does not add any new knowledge and does not make a unique contribution to the body of science. Scholarly manuscripts include support from a body of literature as well as contribute some new knowledge to the body or literature (Sechrist et al., 1987). Thus, publishable scholarly manuscripts include new knowledge, but not knowledge that is so unique and original it does not have a sound foundation in previously established knowledge.

Myth #4: You Need to Complete an Exhaustive Review of the Literature Before You Can Write an Informed Scholarly Manuscript

Most scholarly authors germinate this myth while writing papers for academic classes. One of the purposes of writing papers for a class is to facilitate higher levels of knowledge integration and/or cognitive processing of the specific content by the student. In other words, writing a paper for class is one approach to getting the student to learn content. Writing a paper for class commonly involves a review of the literature that results in students learning and integrating their previously established knowledge in a particular content area. In fact, a requirement of most dissertations is an exhaustive review of the literature in a specific content area. The level of literature review involved in preparing a dissertation results in the student becoming a content expert in that field. The purpose of most scholarly manuscripts, including review manuscripts, is to disseminate new knowledge and not to inform the reader of the entire content area. A scholarly manuscript commonly includes enough review of literature, or background information, to justify the significance and scope of the problem being written about. As well, a scholarly manuscript discusses the meaning of the new knowledge as it relates to previously established knowledge published in the literature. Thus, scholarly authors need an understanding of previous literature in a particular field to justify the issue they are writing about.

THE TITLE: THE FIRST THING AND PERHAPS THE ONLY THING THAT GETS READ

The title is one of the most important components of your scholarly manuscript (Weinert, 2010). A clearly written title assists readers in identifying your manuscript and informs the reader of what knowledge they will gain by reading the manuscript. As well, the title includes key words that can pique the reader's interest. An informative title including key words can assist readers in identifying your manuscript during Internet or electronic searches. By using more descriptive terms in the title such as "balance training exercises" instead of "exercises," readers can more easily identify your manuscript as relevant to their search of the literature. The key words you use in your title tell the reader the variables or concepts you examined and the population in which those variables or concepts were examined.

Scholarly manuscript titles need to be concise and state terms that are used consistently throughout the manuscript. For example, do not include the term "children" in the title and then describe the sample in your manuscript as "infants." The ideal manuscript title has been suggested to be 10 to 12 words in length, although some randomized clinical trials may require longer titles (Pierson, 2004). Most journals set a word or character limit for the manuscripts they publish, so developing a title that presents the main ideas explored in the manuscript is essential. Paiva, Lima, and Paiva (2012) found that data-based manuscripts with short titles describing study results were associated with a greater number of views and citations.

Finally, scholarly manuscript titles need to provide the reader with some insight into what new knowledge the manuscript will provide. The title for a non-data–based manuscript by Hunt, Denieffe, and Gononey (2017) titled, "Burnout and Its Relationship to Empathy in Nursing: A Review of the Literature," clearly informs the reader the manuscript includes a review of manuscripts that examine the relationship between burnout and empathy among nurses. Titles for data-based manuscripts fall into two broad categories: those that describe what was studied, illuminating the design of the study, or those that indicate the results and conclusions of the study (Pierson, 2004; Weinert, 2010). For example, Yayan, Arikan, Saban, Gurarslan Bas, and Ozel Ozcan's (2017) title, "Examination of the Correlation Between Internet Addiction and Social Phobia in Adolescents," indicates that the study design was correlational, conducted among adolescents, and states the variables examined. Notice this title does not disclose the results or conclusions of the study presented in the manuscript. Smoot et al.'s 2017 manuscript title "Potassium Channel Candidate Genes Predict the Development of Secondary Lymphedema Following Breast Cancer Surgery," clearly indicates the results of the study that certain genes predict lymphedema among the population of breast cancer survivors, although this title provides only limited information about the design of the study. Thus, the title of your manuscript informs the reader what new knowledge they will gain by reading your manuscript.

HOW TO WRITE AN ABSTRACT

Like the title, the abstract is commonly one of the first and sometimes the only section of your manuscript that is read. Most readers can access an abstract of a scholarly manuscript online through PubMed or Google Scholar for no charge. To read the full text of a manuscript, the researcher may have to subscribe to the journal, access the journal through their academic institution's library agreement with the publisher, or access the journal through their institution's interlibrary loan agreement with other libraries. This may be part of the reason that some journals require formats for their abstracts that do not "give away" the results of the manuscript. Therefore, like the title, the abstract needs to clearly communicate an idea of what the new knowledge presented in the manuscript is. The content of an abstract aims to answer a number of questions the reader may have after they read the title. These answers briefly inform the reader about (a) why the new knowledge is being presented, (b) the purpose of the manuscript, (c) how the new knowledge was generated, (d) what is the new knowledge, and (e) what the new knowledge means. Abstracts of research studies or data-based manuscripts may be organized within a structured format that roughly corresponds with these questions. This structure organizes the description of the new knowledge into headings including Background (why the new knowledge is being presented), Objectives (the purpose of the manuscript), Methods (how the new knowledge was generated), Results (what is the new knowledge), and Discussion (what the new knowledge means). Abstracts of non-data–based manuscripts may not be formally structured, but they do need to answer these same questions. Finally, the abstract that accompanies your manuscript has implications for reviewing and indexing your manuscript based on the key words and terms you use in the abstract. Choose your key words carefully since these terms will guide readers to (or away from) your manuscript. The more descriptive these key words are, the greater the likelihood that readers searching for literature will find your manuscript appropriate to their search.

WRITING TIP
If you cannot clearly say it in a 300-word abstract then you're probably not going to say it clearly in a 3,000 word manuscript.

The abstract is the first major section of your manuscript that reader swill likely read. So, if your abstract does not hold readers' interest, they will not likely read the rest of your manuscript. Detailed abstracts begin by answering the question, "Why is this new knowledge being presented?" Answering this question commonly involves exploring some unresolved problem the manuscript is attempting to address. This problem is similar to the hook mentioned in Chapter 2, Why Do We (Have to) Write? Depending on the word restrictions of the abstract, answering this question may be implied (not formally stated in short abstracts) or may include several sentences to adequately explain the significance and scope of the problem. Answering this question provides justification to the reader for why the new knowledge is needed.

Next, disclose the purpose of your manuscript early in the abstract. Stating the purpose of the manuscript early in the abstract informs the reader what objective will be met as the result of reading the manuscript. Thus, the reader can judge the relevance of the new knowledge contained in the manuscript and can decide whether to read further. The purpose, also termed the aim or objective, is a clear, concise sentence describing the new knowledge that will be revealed in the manuscript. The purpose of a scholarly manuscript is often stated overtly in a single sentence. For example, "The purpose, aim, or objective of this study or manuscript was to . . ." Examples of purpose statements from data-based and non-data–based scholarly manuscripts are provided in Box 5.1. Notice how these purpose statements are structured the same way by clearly and concisely telling the reader what new knowledge is contained in the manuscript. These purpose statements allude to how the new knowledge was generated, either by a research study (e.g., The purpose of this study . . .) or by combining previously established knowledge (e.g., The purpose of this manuscript is to review collection methods and considerations . . .).

BOX 5.1: EXAMPLES OF PURPOSE STATEMENTS FROM SCHOLARLY MANUSCRIPTS

Data-based manuscripts

The purpose of this study was to examine the relationships of nurse staffing level and work environment with patient adverse events (Cho, Chin, Kim, & Hong, 2016).

The aim of this study was to test and refine a model that identifies which factors are related to home care nurse intentions to remain employed for the next 5 years with their current home care employer organization (Tourangeau, Patterson, Saari, Thomson, & Cranley, 2017).

The objectives of this study were to examine differences in nurse engagement in shared governance across hospitals and to determine the relationship between nurse engagement and patient and nurse outcomes (Kutney-Lee et al., 2016).

Non-data–based manuscripts

Therefore, the aim of this integrative review was to examine the literature related to how open visitation affects the job satisfaction of critical care nurses (Monroe & Wofford, 2017).

This article provides practical advice for coming to emotional terms with rejection and delineates methods for working constructively to address reviewer comments (Conn et al., 2016).

The purpose of this manuscript is to review collection methods and considerations for the acquisition of oral, gut, vaginal, placental, and breast milk microbiome samples in maternal-child health populations (Jordan et al., 2017).

WRITING TIP

When you state the purpose of a manuscript differently, even by changing a single word, you have created a second and competing purpose and have changed the content of the new knowledge you are trying to communicate.

The purpose statement in the abstract needs to be stated consistently throughout the entire manuscript. By consistently I mean EXACTLY THE SAME using the exact same sentence. Early in my career I addressed my tendency to be "creative" when restating the purpose throughout a manuscript by simply cutting and pasting the exact purpose statement whenever I restated the purpose in the document. At times I went as far as to write the purpose on a Post-it Note and attached this note to my computer monitor so I would not forget to state the purpose exactly the same way throughout my manuscript. Consistently stating the purpose throughout the entire manuscript is a pet peeve of most nursing scholars who believe that if an author cannot consistently state the purpose of their manuscript, then the new knowledge presented in the manuscript will likely be inconsistent and difficult to comprehend. The purpose guides the remainder of the manuscript since all these remaining sections are directed toward achieving the purpose. Therefore, the purpose statement answers the reader's second question, "What is the purpose of the manuscript?"

After disclosing the purpose statement, the abstract commonly answers the reader's third question, "How was the new knowledge generated?" New knowledge can be generated through conducting a research study or combining previously generated knowledge in a new way. In a structured abstract of a data-based manuscript, the Methods section includes a description of how the study was conducted, including how the sample was obtained, how the variables were operationalized or measured, how many times the variables were collected, and a description of any intervention that was introduced. After reading the Methods section, the reader has an idea of how the study was conducted to generate the new knowledge. Abstracts of non-data–based manuscripts also provide a brief description of how the new knowledge was developed, although this knowledge is generated by combining previous knowledge in a novel way. In a non-data–based manuscript, this section of the abstract summarizes the previous knowledge and how it is approached from an innovative perspective. Thus, both data-based and non-data–based scholarly manuscript abstracts provide a brief explanation of how the new knowledge was generated.

Following this description of the methodology by which the new knowledge was generated, an abstract answers the question, "What is the new knowledge?" This can be the most challenging section of an abstract to write because the research or combination of previous knowledge commonly results in a lot of new knowledge, all of which cannot be included within the word limitations of an abstract. For example, research studies commonly include new knowledge about the sample and the environment in which the study took place. Similarly, non-data–based manuscripts commonly include a substantial amount of detailed descriptions of previously developed knowledge, all of which cannot be included in an abstract. So how does the author decide what new knowledge to include in the abstract? The answer is to include the new knowledge that addresses the purpose of the manuscript. This section of the abstract clearly and succinctly reveals the new knowledge the author said would be revealed when stating the purpose of the manuscript. For data-based manuscripts, this new knowledge is commonly supported with statistical findings that may include descriptive (frequencies, means, standard deviations, etc.) as well as inferential analysis (r, R^2, t, f, etc.). As well, you may wish to indicate the level of statistical significance that you set *a priori* for these inferential statistical analyses. Authors convey statistical significance in various ways. Some state the analysis was "statistically significant" or "significant." Others present the inferential statistic with the probability of type I error for the statistic (p <). While some authors state the results of the inferential analysis as differences, correlations, predictors, and the like followed by a *p*-level, they assume the reader will understand that using those words implies statistical significance. For non-data–based manuscripts, this section of the abstract also presents a brief description of the new knowledge that addresses the purpose of the manuscript. Again, many authors struggle with writing this section of a non-data–based abstract, because they commonly generate a lot of new knowledge in the manuscript. Staying focused on addressing the purpose of the manuscript will direct you in writing this section of the abstract.

Once you inform the reader of the new knowledge that is provided in the manuscript, the final portion of the abstract frames the new knowledge or informs the reader about what the new knowledge means. For data-based manuscripts, this portion of the abstract is commonly labeled Discussion, Conclusions, or Clinical Implications. Addressing the question of what the new knowledge means is based on the initial portion of the abstract that provides the rationale supporting why the new knowledge is needed or what problem needs to be addressed through generating this knowledge. In other words, this section tells the reader how the new knowledge contributes toward addressing the problem that justified engaging in the generating the knowledge in the first place. The author of the manuscript may also choose to describe how the new knowledge extends the current knowledge in the literature, directs future research, refines a theoretical framework, or can provide evidence to support clinical practice. The final section of the abstract directs the reader how to use the new knowledge presented in the manuscript to address some unresolved problem. This new knowledge may not completely resolve the problem but provides some new knowledge contributing to a future resolution of the problem.

The following is an example of the importance of including a section in the abstract explaining what the new knowledge means. I had conducted a study examining the efficacy of a topical gel to reduce joint pain, and I was asked to share the abstract of my preliminary findings with the marketing department of the company that manufactured the gel. The results section of the abstract reported that "the sample's pain rating within 10 minutes of applying the gel to the painful joint, changed nonsignificantly (p>.05) from a rating of 4 to 2 on the 10-point visual analog scale used to measure pain." I failed to provide a conclusion in the abstract about what this new knowledge meant. A week later I read on the company's website that, citing my abstract, the gel reduced pain by 50% and can "cut your pain in half." At this point I realized I needed to indicate in my original abstract that this nonsignificant change in pain appears to merit further study to determine the clinical importance of the findings.

WRITING TIP
Creating a document is much more difficult then editing a pre-existing document. Whenever possible use previously written documents as the starting point for writing new documents.

Abstracts of data-based and non-data–based scholarly manuscripts need to address the same five questions: (a) why the new knowledge is being presented; (b) what is the purpose of the manuscript; (c) how was the new knowledge was generated; (d) what is the new knowledge; and (e) what does the new knowledge mean? Exhibit 5.1 presents a template following this format for constructing an abstract of a data-based scholarly manuscript.

Exhibit 5.2 is a template for a non–data-based scholarly manuscript. These templates are similar because all scholarly manuscripts involve presenting new knowledge. New knowledge can be based on the presentation of new data analysis (data-based manuscript) or the presentation or combination of previously established data in some new way (non–data-based manuscript).

The process of creating an abstract is similar to the process involved when creating a scholarly manuscript. This process involves creating

---

EXHIBIT 5.1: TEMPLATE FOR AN ABSTRACT OF A DATA-BASED SCHOLARLY MANUSCRIPT

Title: Include the variables or concepts you examined and the population in which the variables or concepts were examined.
Type of titles:

1. Describe what was studied by illuminating the design of the study.

2. Indicate the results and conclusions of the study.

Background (Why is the new knowledge being presented?): State the problem that the new knowledge will address. Present this problem in terms of the scope of the problem or how many individuals are affected, the significance of a problem, or the negative impact of the problem on money (excessive costs or lost actual or potential revenue), increasing morbidity or mortality, and/or deteriorating quality of life.

Objectives (What is the purpose of the manuscript?): State a single sentence beginning with "The purpose, aim, or objective of this study was to. . . ."

Methods (How was new knowledge generated?): Describe how the study was conducted including how the sample was obtained, how the variables were operationalized or measured, how many times the variables were collected, and any intervention that was introduced.

(continued)

EXHIBIT 5.1: TEMPLATE FOR AN ABSTRACT OF A DATA-BASED
SCHOLARLY MANUSCRIPT (*continued*)

Results (What is the new knowledge?): Present descriptive data
(count, frequencies, percentages, mean, standard deviations,
etc.) and statistical analysis (χ^2, t, f, r, β, etc.), which address
the purpose, aim, or objective. Indicate if these statistics are
statistically significant in the text or by indicating the probability
of type I error ($p<$) of the statistic.

Discussion (What does the new knowledge mean?): Tell the
reader how the new knowledge contributes toward addressing
the problem mentioned in the Background section. Explain to the
reader how this new knowledge will contribute to saving money,
decreasing death and illness, and improving quality of life. This
contribution may be in the form of supporting future research,
validating or refuting knowledge in the literature, developing
a theoretical, and/or providing evidence to support clinical
practice.

EXHIBIT 5.2: TEMPLATE FOR AN ABSTRACT OF A
NON-DATA–BASED SCHOLARLY MANUSCRIPT

Title: Include the variables or concepts that you combined and the
new knowledge that resulted. You may include the population to
which the new knowledge is relevant.

(Why is the new knowledge being presented?) State the problem
that the new knowledge will address. Present this problem in
terms of the scope of the problem, or how many individuals are
affected and the significance of a problem, or the negative impact
of the problem on money (excessive costs or lost actual or potential
revenue), increasing morbidity or mortality, and/or deteriorating
quality of life.

(What is the purpose of the manuscript?) State a single sentence
beginning with "The purpose, aim, or objective of this manuscript
is to. . . ."

(How was new knowledge generated?) Describe how the study
was conducted including how the sample was obtained, how
the variables were operationalized or measured, how many
times the variables were collected, and any intervention that was
introduced.

(*continued*)

EXHIBIT 5.2: TEMPLATE FOR AN ABSTRACT OF A
NON-DATA–BASED SCHOLARLY MANUSCRIPT (*continued*)

(What is the new knowledge?) Present descriptive data (count, frequencies, percentages, mean, standard deviations, etc.) and statistical analysis (χ^2, t, f, r, β, etc.), which address the purpose, aim, or objective. Indicate if these statistics are statistically significant in the text or by indicating the probability of type I error ($p<$) of the statistic.

(What does the new knowledge mean?) Tell the reader how the new knowledge contributes toward addressing the problem you mentioned in the Background section. Explain to the reader how this new knowledge will contribute to saving money, decreasing death and illness, and improving quality of life. This contribution may be in the form of supporting future research, validating or refuting knowledge in the literature, developing a theoretical, and/or providing evidence to support clinical practice.

---

and then revising a number of preliminary drafts before the final version is produced. Many authors ask when, during the development of a scholarly manuscript, is the best time to compose the abstract? To answer this question, I would like to point out some resources you may have previously written that can help you write your abstract. Composing an abstract is rarely the first step in developing a document intended to communicate new knowledge. Commonly, composing an abstract is preceded by a written proposal for the project, analysis of data or previously developed knowledge, and interpretation of the new knowledge, all of which contribute to a preliminary draft of a manuscript. Consequently, an abstract of a scholarly manuscript is much easier to write once the preliminary draft of the manuscript is completed. Once you have written the preliminary draft of your scholarly manuscript you can "copy and paste" sections from the main document to provide preliminary versions of sections of the abstract. For example, the author can copy the purpose statement from the main document and paste the exact statement into the abstract. This copy- and-paste approach is similar when generating the content to address the other sections of the abstract. Content that answers the question "Why is this new knowledge being presented?" can be copied from the introduction or background of the draft manuscript and pasted into the proper section of the abstract. Other sections of the abstract can be developed in a similar way by copying the methodology, results, and conclusions sections from the first draft of the manuscript and pasting them into the abstract. This copy and paste approach will result in a rough, long, first draft of your abstract. Once you have this first draft "written," you can begin the process of revising the content to clearly and succinctly communicate the new knowledge you have discovered.

There are advantages and disadvantages to writing your abstract by this copy-and-paste approach. First, this approach commonly results in the abstract's first draft being long and exceeding the word limits of the instructions. However, since this lengthy first draft of your abstract is copied from previously developed documents, this approach results in consistent use of terms between these documents and the first draft of the abstract. Second, this copy-and-paste approach requires you to have written a preliminary draft of the scholarly manuscript.

On occasion, you may need to generate an abstract before you have completed a first draft of a manuscript. Nursing scholars commonly submit abstracts for presentations at professional meetings before completing a manuscript that communicates the new knowledge. In these instances, without a first draft of a manuscript, there are likely other preliminary documents that can be used for content to populate the abstract using the copy and paste approach. These other documents include the project proposal, an institutional review board (IRB) application, or a similar, previously developed abstract. A third limitation when using this copy-and-paste approach to developing the first draft of your abstract is that you may have developed an emotional or intellectual attachment to sentences and phrases that are appropriate in the manuscript but too long for your abstract. I am guilty of "falling in love" with some sentences and paragraphs that I believe perfectly convey the points I want to make. I have great difficulty revising these so-called perfect sentences and paragraphs. When that happens, I consult an external reviewer, who I sometimes refer to as "Shiva," to help me revise the sentences and paragraphs I thought were unassailable. A final limitation of the copy-and-paste approach is that the first draft of the abstract will likely be disorganized, lacking a clear logical flow and smooth transitions between sentences and paragraphs. Using this approach will require editing the content of the first draft to meet the word count limitations and to communicate the new knowledge clearly and succinctly.

Once you have written a first draft of an abstract you have to decrease or prune the content in order to meet the word count limitations. Pruning an abstract is like pruning tomato plants. When I prune my tomato plants, I decide which branches are not directly contributing to the overall purpose of the plant and which branches are, to varying degrees, essential to the purpose of the plant in producing tomatoes. When deciding what to prune from the first draft of an abstract, you must constantly decide if the content is essential to the purpose of the abstract, clearly and succinctly communicating the new knowledge. Exhibit 5.3 is the first draft of an abstract I created by copying-and-pasting sections of a previously written proposal and sections of a manuscript draft. This first draft of the abstract is 646 words long with 10 citations and references to appendices.

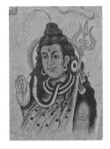

Shiva, the Hindu God of destruction.
Source: Courtesy of Antoine Taveneaux

EXHIBIT 5.3: FIRST DRAFT OF AN ABSTRACT COPIED AND PASTED FROM THE FIRST DRAFT OF A MANUSCRIPT

Word Count = 640 plus 10 references
The effect of Theraworx Relief™ on night-time leg cramps and associated symptoms among older adults.

Night-time leg cramps (NLC) is a musculoskeletal disorder related to magnesium deficiency presenting as sudden, episodic, persistent, painful, involuntary contractions of the leg muscles at night. Approximately 33% of individuals age 50 years and older report NLC resulting in the associated symptoms of poor sleep quality, poor quality of life, and depression. Theraworx Relief™ is a topical therapy containing magnesium sulfate and anecdotal evidence indicates this therapy reduces leg cramps among athletes.

No treatment for NLC has been proven both safe and effective [1]. Magnesium is a critical element in numerous metabolic reactions and in muscle functioning **[7]** with magnesium deficiency leading to neural excitability and muscle cramping [8]. The administration of oral magnesium salts has been shown to be effective in the treatment of pregnancy-associated leg cramps [9]. The results of a systematic review of randomized controlled trials with a meta-analysis in the area reported no clear efficacy of orally administered magnesium salts on leg cramps [10]. To date no study has examined the impact of topically applied magnesium on frequency and severity of night-time cramps and associated symptoms. Theraworx Relief™ is a topical homeopathic therapy that contains magnesium sulfate and has anecdotal evidence supporting the efficacy of this therapy to reduce leg cramps among athletes (https://innergysport.com). **The purpose of this study was to determine the effect of Theraworx Relief™ on the frequency and severity of night-time leg cramps and associated symptoms, including sleep quality, quality of life, and depression.**
50 subjects who reported experiencing NLC at least three times per week volunteered to participate in a 4-week double blind clinical trial evaluating the efficacy of Theraworx Relief™ and a placebo condition. Individuals were enrolled if they reported experiencing night-time cramps and spasms

Since this abstract was "written" by cut-and-paste from other documents the references are not ordered.

Notice how the key purpose statements stays the same in all versions of the abstract.

(continued)

EXHIBIT 5.3: FIRST DRAFT OF AN ABSTRACT COPIED AND PASTED FROM THE FIRST DRAFT OF A MANUSCRIPT (*continued*)

(see Appendix G) on average at least three times per week. Recruitment efforts included various targeted methods (newspaper, flyers in pharmacies and physician offices, social media, sleep disorder support groups, etc.). Individuals were excluded from the study if they were pregnant, have been previously diagnosed with a non-RLS sleep disorder, previously diagnosed with schizophrenia or any other neurological disorder. Subjects self-reported their sleep quality, quality of life, and depression upon entering into the study (baseline), following 2 weeks of no treatment (post control) and again following 2 weeks of either topically applying Theraworx Relief™ or a placebo (post treatment). In addition, subjects completed a daily diary indicating the frequency and severity of night-time cramps, which were collapsed into weekly intervals. During the 2-week treatment period all subjects were instructed to apply their assigned topical treatment to their legs bilaterally before retiring to bed in the evening and use additional amounts of the topical treatment if leg cramping occurred. At baseline, the 24 individuals who were assigned to receive the placebo were similar on all outcome measures and most demographic variables to the 25 individuals who received the Theraworx Relief™. Following the trial, 60% of the group receiving the Theraworx Relief™ claimed a benefit of the treatment, while 41% of the subjects receiving the placebo claimed a benefit of the treatment ($\chi^2 = 1.65$, $p = 20$). Repeated measures ANOVA analysis indicated that subjects who received Theraworx Relief™ exhibited statistically significant declines in the frequency of cramps and the severity by frequency of cramps between week 1 and week 4 of the study. Subjects receiving the placebo did not exhibit a change in these measures between weeks 1 and 4. Subjects receiving Theraworx Relief™ exhibited significant ($p < 0.05$) improvements between baseline and post treatment and post control and post treatment on the outcomes measures of sleep quality, quality of life, and depression. The subjects receiving the placebo did not significantly change as a result of their treatment on any of these measures during these study intervals.

Individuals who experienced NLC three or more times per week reported a significant reduction in leg cramps and improved their quality of life, depression, and sleep quality as a result of nightly use of Theraworx Relief™.

Exhibit 5.4 is an abstract of the same manuscript decreased to 300 words, and Exhibit 5.5 presents an abstract of the manuscript consisting of 150 words. Notice there are certain essential sentences or content that are preserved in all versions of the abstract. These sentences in all three versions of the abstract are needed to communicate the new knowledge. The purpose is stated consistently in all three versions of the abstract. Within the methods section, the sample size, data collection intervals, description of the treatment and placebo condition, and the outcome variables are preserved in all three versions. The Results section in all three versions clearly states how the outcome variables changed, thereby addressing the purpose. Finally, the application of the results is preserved in the discussion of all three versions that the independent variable (Theraworx Relief™) decreased night-time leg cramps and improved the associated symptoms of sleep quality, quality of life, and depression.

EXHIBIT 5.4: SECOND DRAFT OF AN ABSTRACT

Word count = 300

The effect of Theraworx Relief™ on night-time leg cramps and associated symptoms among older adults

Background: Night-time leg cramps (NLC) is a musculoskeletal disorder related to magnesium deficiency presenting as sudden, episodic, persistent, painful, involuntary contractions of the leg muscles at night. Approximately 33% of older adults, age 50 years and older, report NLC resulting in the associated symptoms of poor sleep quality, poor quality of life, and depression. Theraworx Relief™ is a topical therapy containing magnesium that has been shown to reduce leg cramps among athletes.

Purpose: **The purpose of this study was to determine the effect of Theraworx Relief™ on the frequency and severity of night-time leg cramps and associated symptoms, including sleep quality, quality of life and depression.**

Methods: Fifty older adults reporting NLC at least three times per week participated in a 4-week double blind clinical trial. Subjects' sleep quality, quality of life, and depression were measured upon entering into the study (baseline), following 2 weeks of no treatment (post control) and again following 2 weeks of either topically applying Theraworx Relief™ or a placebo (post treatment). Subjects completed a daily diary indicating the frequency and severity of their night-time cramps, which were collapsed into weekly intervals. During the 2-week treatment period all subjects applied their assigned topical treatment to their legs before retiring in the evening.

The EXACT same purpose statement

(continued)

EXHIBIT 5.4: SECOND DRAFT OF AN ABSTRACT (*continued*)

Results: Subjects who received Theraworx Relief™ exhibited significant ($p < 0.05$) declines in the frequency of cramps and the severity between week 1 and week 4 of the study. Subjects receiving Theraworx Relief™ exhibited significant ($p < 0.05$) improvements on measures of sleep quality, quality of life, and depression. Subjects receiving the placebo did not change any outcome measures between weeks 1 and 4.

Discussion: Individuals who experienced NLC reported a reduction in leg cramps and improved their sleep quality, quality of life and depression and as a result of nightly use of Theraworx Relief™.

EXHIBIT 5.5: THIRD DRAFT OF AN ABSTRACT

Word count = 150
The effect of Theraworx Relief™ on night-time leg cramps and associated symptoms among older adults

The EXACT same purpose statement →

Purpose: The purpose of this study was to determine the effect of Theraworx Relief™ on the frequency and severity of night-time leg cramps (NLC) and associated symptoms, including sleep quality, quality of life, and depression.

Methods: Fifty older adults self-reported their sleep quality, quality of life, and depression at baseline, following 2-weeks of no treatment (post control), and again following 2 weeks of either topically applying Theraworx Relief™ or a placebo (post treatment). NLC were reported daily and collapsed into weekly intervals. During the treatment period all subjects applied their assigned topical treatment to their legs before retiring in the evening.

Results: Subjects who received Theraworx Relief™ reduced ($p < 0.05$) their NLC and improved their sleep quality, quality of life, and depression. Subjects receiving the placebo did not change any outcome measures.

Discussion: Nightly use of Theraworx Relief™ reduces leg cramps and improves sleep quality, quality of life and depression.

CONCLUSION

I began this chapter describing a struggle I had early in my career in creating an abstract that communicated new knowledge in a clear and succinct format. This early struggle may have been based on some myths I fostered that scholarly manuscripts needed to have broad implications, wide appeal with distinctive new knowledge based on an exhaustive review of the literature. This chapter describes how the title of the manuscript informs the reader of what knowledge they will gain by reading the manuscript. After reading the title, the abstract provides answers the reader may have about why the new knowledge is being presented, what is the purpose of the manuscript, how the new knowledge was generated, what is the new knowledge, and what does the new knowledge mean. Further, I described how to write a first draft of an abstract using a copy and paste approach from previously developed documents. Finally, I presented an example of writing a first draft of an abstract using the copy-and-paste approach and illustrated how to prune the content of this first draft to a 300- and 150-word final abstract that describes the new knowledge generated.

REFERENCES

Cho, E., Chin, D. L., Kim, S., & Hong, O. (2016). The relationships of nurse staffing level and work environment with patient adverse events. *Journal of Nursing Scholarship, 48*(1), 74–82. doi:10.1111/jnu.12183

Conn, V. S., Zerwic, J., Jefferson, U., Anderson, C. M., Killion, C. M., Smith, C. E., . . . Loya, J. (2016). Normalizing rejection. *Western Journal of Nursing Research, 38*(2), 137–154. doi:10.1177/0193945915589538

Hunt, P. A., Denieffe, S., & Gooney, M. (2017). Burnout and its relationship to empathy in nursing: A review of the literature. *Journal of Research in Nursing, 22*(1–2), 7–22.

Jordan, S., Baker, B., Dunn, A., Edwards, S., Ferranti, E., Mutic, A. D., . . . Rodriguez, J. (2017). Maternal-child microbiome: Specimen collection, storage, and implications for research and practice. *Nursing Research, 66*(2), 175–183. doi:10.1097/NNR.0000000000000201

Juhl, N., & Norman, V. L. (1989). Writing an effective abstract. *Applied Nursing Research, 2*(4), 189–191.

Kutney-Lee, A., Germack, H., Hatfield, L., Kelly, S., Maguire, P., Dierkes, A., . . . Aiken, L. H. (2016). Nurse engagement in shared governance and patient and nurse outcomes. *Journal of Nursing Adminstration, 46*(11), 605–612. doi:10.1097/NNA.0000000000000412

Monroe, M., & Wofford, L. (2017). Open visitation and nurse job satisfaction: An integrative review. *Journal of Clinical Nursing, 26*(23–24), 4868–4876. doi:10.1111/jocn.13919

Paiva, C. E., Lima, J. P., & Paiva, B. S. (2012). Articles with short titles describing the results are cited more often. *Clinics (Sao Paulo), 67*(5), 509–513.

Pender, N. J., & Pender, A. R. (1985). Attitudes, subjective norms, and intentions to engage in health behaviors. *Nursing Research, 35*(1), 15–18.

Pender, N. J., Walker, S. N., Sechrist, K. R., & Frank-Stromborg, M. (1990). Predicting health-promoting lifestyles in the workplace. *Nursing Research, 39*(6), 326–332.

Pierson, D. J. (2004). How to write an abstract that will be accepted for presentation at a national meeting. *Respiratory Care, 49*(10), 1206–1212.

Sechrist, K. R., Walker, S. N., & Pender, N. J. (1987). Development and psychometric evaluation of the exercise benefits/barriers scale. *Research in Nursing & Health, 10*(6), 357–365.

Smoot, B., Kober, K. M., Paul, S. M., Levine, J. D., Abrams, G., Mastick, J., ... Miaskowski, C. A. (2017). Potassium channel candidate genes predict the development of secondary lymphedema following breast cancer surgery. *Nursing Research, 66*(2), 85–94.

Tourangeau, A. E., Patterson, E., Saari, M., Thomson, H., & Cranley, L. (2017). Work-related factors influencing home care nurse intent to remain employed. *Health Care Management Review, 42*(1), 87–97. doi:10.1097/HMR.0000000000000093

Walker, S. N., Volkan, K., Sechrist, K. R., & Pender, N. J. (1988). Health-promoting life styles of older adults: Comparisons with young and middle-aged adults, correlates and patterns. *Advances in Nursing Science, 11*(1), 76–90.

Weil, B. H. (1970). Standards for writing abstracts. *Journal of the Association for Information Science and Technology, 21*(5), 351–357.

Weinert, C. (2010). Are all abstracts created equal?? *Applied Nursing Research, 23*(2), 106–109. doi:10.1016/j.apnr.2008.06.003

Yayan, E. H., Arikan, D., Saban, F., Gurarslan Bas, N., & Ozel Ozcan, O. (2017). Examination of the correlation between Internet addiction and social phobia in adolescents. *Western Journal of Nursing Research, 39*(9), 1240–1254. doi:10.1177/0193945916665820

CHAPTER 6

WRITING FOR EMPLOYMENT: THE PROCESS OF SECURING A JOB IN ACADEMIA

Robert Topp

PERSONAL STORY

"More school? You must be out of your mind!" That was my initial thought when my dissertation advisor recommended I apply for a post-doctoral fellowship. My next thought was, "Are you trying to tell me you didn't do a good job preparing me for a job in academia?" After I thought about it, I realized that completing an additional 2 years of post-doctoral training would probably provide me with additional skills to jump-start my program of research at a research-intensive college of nursing. I skimmed the description of the post-doctoral program and the application process. Up to this point in my career, the nursing staff jobs I had applied for involved filling in the blanks on an application and completing a two-step interview. Step one was meeting with the human resources department to ensure I qualified for the position and to explain benefits and salary. The second step commonly involved meeting with the unit director and maybe one or two other nursing staff for an hour to discuss the job qualifications and duties of the position. I thought the application materials for the post-doctoral position were straight forward and requested that I include a brief statement of my professional and research goals and three letters of reference. I sat down and "knocked out" my professional goals, including conducting research that examined how physical and psychological functioning could be improved through engaging in regular physical activity.

The post-doctoral position was my first interview for an academic position. I reviewed the interview schedule and was surprised that would be meeting with 15 different people starting at 7:30 a.m. with breakfast and ending at 6:30 p.m. with dinner at the faculty club with the program director. My interview was going to be 11 hours long and included an hour-long scholarly presentation of my dissertation. By the time I arrived at the faculty club, my new Galen plaid interview suit that included a starched button-down white shirt with matching yellow paisley tie and suspenders (this was the late '80s), was starting to feel like an oxen's yoke. I could only vaguely recall the salad I had for lunch that was inadequate for most rodents, and I was kicking myself for not eating the puck-sized roll that accompanied my meal. I sat down with the program director (a gregarious academician that could be easily confused with a part-time mall Santa) and he began our meeting by saying "I bet you have had an interesting day. I insist you have three fingers of my private stock, 12-year old scotch." (I hate scotch. It always tastes like something I would use to start the briquettes at the barbeque.) After sipping while trying not to consume this hydrocarbon-based fluid, the director started with, "How do you see our training program aligning with your professional goal?" I started to think that the first 11 hours of the day were to soften me up and now the real interview was about to begin. Doing my homework paid off! I recalled the literature I had skimmed about how the training program offered access to five large ongoing research projects, each examining some aspect of chronic diseases associated with aging. I began to wonder if the director had read my application because he never asked about my professional goals or research. The one thing he repeatedly asked about was how I had mentioned in my application that I had been employed as a research assistant on a project that examined the effect of exercise on physical and cognitive functioning among older adults. After some BS'ing, which the scotch likely allowed the program director to tolerate, I finally was able to pivot and started to explain how pursuing my research could contribute to the ongoing research project that was examining how different levels of exercise affect blood glucose levels among type II diabetics. After some affirming nods, I then described how I could contribute to the objectives of the overall training program and achieve the aims of one of the research projects. Once I was able to match my abilities with the objectives of the training program, the director seemed satisfied and I was eventually hired. I finally finished my drink and commented how "smooth" it was.

INTRODUCTION

In hindsight, it is easy to pick out the many errors I made on my way to securing my first academic appointment. The purpose of this chapter is to describe the general process of locating, applying for, interviewing, and negotiating an academic position. Various steps in this process involve creating written documents. It is important that you write down information in order to more clearly conceptualize your thinking. I will present a number of steps including locating, applying for, interviewing, and negotiating an academic position. These steps take you from identifying a position that aligns with your skills, preparation, personal and professional goals, to negotiating and securing an academic position.

FIVE STEPS FOR ACQUIRING AN ACADEMIC POSITION

Step 1: Deciding What You Want to Be When You Grow Up

I have been asked this question repeatedly my entire life. Whenever I gave an answer of a specific occupation, such as firefighter, astronaut, rodeo clown, or nurse, there was always the inevitable follow-up question, "Why do you want to do that?" My rationale to justify pursuing a particular occupation might be to drive the fire truck with the siren, to float weightless in space, to wear interesting clothes to work, or to help people feel better. The truth is very few people know what they want to do when they grow up even after they are grown up. I continue to ask myself some important questions like, "Am I making a contribution? Is the world a better place because of me? Am I doing as well as my peers?" The best answer I have come up with so far is, "When I grow up I want to be happy." Whenever I give this answer no one asks for rationale or asks me "Why do you want to do that?"

> **WRITING LIFE TIP**
> If what you do everyday doesn't make you happy, then you have to ask yourself why do you keep doing it?

Do not be seduced into dismissing my answer to this question because it is simplistic. An essential goal that is pursued at every age is to be happy, content, or self-actualized (Robertson, 2016). As an adult, the challenge is figuring out how to achieve this goal while maintaining employment since many of us do not have the resources to pursue our goals without generating income through working. The first thing to write down when beginning your pursuit of an academic position are the job activities that will contribute to your happiness. Perhaps you find happiness in teaching students, conducting research, advancing the department or profession through service, or practicing nursing. Writing down components of an academic position that contribute to your happiness will help you to identify a satisfying position.

Jobs in academia offer a wide variety of opportunities, roles, and duties. Academic positions in nursing may include varying amounts of teaching, research, service, administrative, and/or practice responsibilities. These areas of academic responsibility are consistent with the four aspects of scholarship described by Boyer (1990), which include the scholarship of teaching, discovery, integration, and application, respectively.

I like to think of an academic position as a pie with each section of the pie indicating a percentage of time dedicated to a particular area of responsibility. For example, Figure 6.1 is a typical academic appointment for a tenure-track assistant professor at a research-intensive university with 50% of the appointment dedicated to teaching, 30% to scholarship/research and 20% to service. Figure 6.2 represents the percentage of time dedicated to teaching, scholarship, and service for a non-tenure-track clinical instructor at a teaching-intensive institution. Notice the tenure-track appointment includes a larger percentage of time dedicated to scholarship/research and service while almost all of the non-tenure-track clinical or educational appointment is dedicated to teaching.

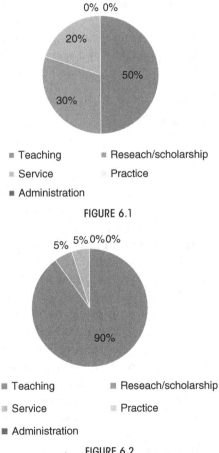

FIGURE 6.1

FIGURE 6.2

So, you will have completed the first step in securing an academic position when you are able to write down job activities that will make you happy within an academic position. This includes a congruent amount of teaching, research, service, and practice responsibilities. If the teaching, research, service, administration, and/or practice activities within academic nursing do not seem to make you happy, then stop reading this chapter, place this book on your bookshelf, and reconsider your choice of vocations because you will not be happy in academic nursing.

Step 2: Find a Position That Will Make You Happy

Once you have decided on a mix of job responsibilities that will contribute to your happiness, you will need to find an academic position that requires you to engage in those types of responsibilities. Qualified nursing faculty are in short supply in the United States, so there is an abundant number of open faculty positions. In 2016, the American Association of Colleges of Nursing (AACN) reported a total of 1,567 nursing faculty vacancies across the country. Besides these vacancies, schools cited the need to create an additional 133 faculty positions to accommodate student demand. The data show a national nurse faculty vacancy rate of 7.9%. Most of the vacancies (92.8%) were faculty positions requiring or preferring a doctoral degree (AACN, 2018). This good news is also bad news because this faculty shortage means that most colleges of nursing are understaffed by faculty who are asked to take on "overloaded" work assignments.

Identifying open nursing faculty positions can be done using a variety of strategies. The challenge will be finding an open nursing faculty position that that includes roles and responsibilities that will make you happy. The four most common approaches to identifying open faculty positions are professional search firms, professional journals or publications, professional networking, and searching specific colleges or universities. Professional search firms or "head hunters" have a contract with a school to identify individuals who are qualified for academic positions. These firms, through a variety of means, advertise the open position, recruit potential candidates, and may initially screen candidates and identify a sample of individuals who have expressed an interest and meet some threshold of qualifications for the position. Accessing the services of these professional search firms is commonly free of charge to the individual seeking a position. However, some of these firms provide interview coaching, resume building, and other services to the individual job seeker on a fee-for-service basis. Larger search firms commonly have search filters on their websites for positions with specific job requirements in specific states.

Advertisements in professional journals or publications are another source for finding open faculty positions. For example, the *Chronicle of Higher Education* (*The Chronicle*) lists a large number of open faculty positions across disciplines and areas of the country. Printed and electronic editions of journals that focus on a nursing specialty commonly include open position announcements for faculty who have expertise in that specialty. For example, *Nursing Research* commonly includes open academic and clinical nursing positions with a research focus, while the *Journal of Pediatric Nursing* includes a link to open academic positions requiring content expertise in pediatric nursing. These advertisements in professional journals or publications are often placed by search firms and specific colleges or universities.

Professional networking to identify open nursing faculty positions can be done at professional meetings or conferences as well as through professional networking websites. Attending the vendor area of a nursing professional meetings facilitates direct face-to-face contact with representatives of colleges and universities who have open academic positions. I have observed short, informal interviews take place at these professional meetings, so if you attend a professional meeting looking for available positions, be ready to engage in an "informal interview" including sharing your curriculum vitae and articulating your unique contributions to the mission and goals of the institution. More recently, professional networking websites including LinkedIn, Research Gate, Facebook, and others have emerged and can identify open academic positions that match the qualifications you list on your profile (see Chapter 9, Difficult Documents). Finally, many schools and colleges of nursing have open positions posted on their institutional webpage.

Once you have identified an open position, **closely read the position description.** Carefully determine if you possess the qualifications of the position. Sometimes these qualifications are quantifiable and specific, for example, possessing a minimum of 5 years of teaching experience in a nursing undergraduate program; or they may be vague and broad, for example, possessing an established record of nationally recognized research productivity and extramural funding. Regardless of the level of detail of the qualifications, you need to write down how you meet or exceed each of the qualifications listed on the position description. Writing down how you meet or exceed the qualifications and evidence that supports your ability to perform the duties and responsibilities will indicate whether you are eligible. Formatting your qualifications in a table format will provide an outline for developing your application letter for the position. If you cannot write down how your qualifications and experiences match at least some of the position requirements and provide some examples of your experience in performing the role and responsibilities of the posted position, then do not apply for the position—you will be wasting your time.

In addition to reading the position description, also **read the institution's mission/vision/values statements**. These statements tend to be broad, all-encompassing and, therefore, vague (e.g., Marquette University aspires to be, and to be recognized, among the most innovative and accomplished Catholic and Jesuit universities in the world, promoting the greater glory of God and the well-being of humankind; Marquette University, 2018). Also, become familiar with the academic unit's strategic plan, goals, or objectives. These unit goal statements have been developed to contribute to the mission/vision/values statements and are stated more quantitatively (e.g., Strategic Goal II: The University of Iowa College of Nursing will intensify the quality and quantity of research and scholarship to achieve top 10 ranking by NIH; The University of Iowa, 2018). In your application letter and throughout the interview process you will need to describe how you intend to contribute to the academic unit's strategic plan, goals, or objectives. You do not need to explain how you will contribute to every component of the academic unit's strategic plan

WRITING TIP

Check for spelling, grammar and content errors in your application letter. The content accuracy of this letter provides a first impression of your attention to detail to your prospective employer.

or every goal, but you do need to be able to describe how you intend to contribute to some of these goals. A successful job seeker can clearly articulate how the institution will benefit and move toward achieving their goals because of hiring the job seeker. Developing a written matrix of how, based on your qualifications and experiences, you will contribute to the institution's strategic plan, goals, and objectives will also assist you in developing your application letter.

Exhibit 6.1 presents a fictional job posting for an academic nursing position with comments about the important information in the posting. This job posting begins with a brief description of the school of nursing, how it is organized within the university, and the type of academic programs offered within the school. The next section presents the principal duties and responsibilities, or what the day-to-day role of the position involves. Following the fictional job posting is a list of required and preferred qualifications of applicants. Finally, the posting instructs the applicant what to do next if they are interested in applying for the position; submit a cover letter and CV to a specific contact person.

EXHIBIT 6.1: JOB POSTING FOR AN ACADEMIC NURSING POSITION

Tenure Track Faculty Position Post

Assistant Professor

The School of Nursing (SON) at Bob University is seeking applicants for several 10-month tenure-track faculty positions beginning in fall [year]. **The SON is committed to BU and the College of Health and Human Services' mission of excellence in teaching. The SON also strives to extend knowledge through research and to prepare caring and competent professionals to enhance health and quality of life within the global community.**

The SON is one of four schools within the College of Health and Human Services at Bob University. The other schools include Exercise Science, Social Work, and Health Education and Promotion. The SON offers BSN, 2nd Degree BSN, BSN 2+2 degree, Collaborative BSN degree, BSN completion, online RN-BSN degree, MSN degrees in Adult-Gero CNS, Adult-Gero Primary Care NP, and Nursing Education. As well, The SON anticipates admitting its inaugural class of DNP students in fall [next year].

Callout: Notice the duration of the appointment.

Callout: Notice this is a tenure-track position.

Callout: Referral to the institution's mission and the School's strategic goals.

Callout: Notice the SON is within a larger College that includes health professions but no clinical health professions.

(continued)

EXHIBIT 6.1: JOB POSTING FOR AN ACADEMIC NURSING POSITION (*continued*)

Principal Duties and Responsibilities

All teaching responsibilities.

Teach graduate-level and undergraduate-level courses as assigned by the department or school.

Assign and submit grades according to university schedules.

Host regular office hours at times that are convenient for students.

Offer academic advising to students.

Does NOT say engage in independent research trajectory, lead a research team, submit for extramural funding, publish and/or present findings.

Engage in pursuits that will enable you to remain up-to-date in your respective disciplines.

Seems to suggest practice and to maintain advanced practice certification.

Engage in pursuits to help further contribute to the body of knowledge in your respective disciplines, and/or to research interdisciplinary implications.

All appear to be service to the School, College, or University.

Serve as a member of search committees for new faculty members, departmental committees, and other university service committees.

Support university-wide activities such as orientation, convocation, student registration, and commencement.

Attend scheduled departmental meetings and functions.

Provide supportive services to the department, college, and/or university, as necessary.

This is a catch-all that means anything the department chair deems important could be assigned to you.

Perform departmental duties as necessary.

The faculty are represented by a collective bargaining unit.

This position is covered under the collective bargaining agreement between [university] and the [university] Chapter of the American Association of University Professors, which settles all matters regarding wages, hours, benefits, and other employment terms and conditions.

Qualifications

They do not stipulate the doctoral degree is a PhD or DNP and the doctoral degree is nursing is NOT required.

Required: **Doctoral degree** from an accredited program prior to start date. Three years of clinical experience as a master's-prepared nurse practitioner in **Psychiatric-Mental Health, Family Health, or Obstetrics / Maternal Child, or Adult-Gerontology**

These are the areas of clinical expertise they are interested in recruiting. Notice no previous academic teaching experience is required but it is preferred.

Preferred Qualifications: Teaching experience in an undergraduate program. Experience with online course development and delivery. Scholarly productivity in the form of publications and presentations

These are preferred, not essential qualifications. Notice how these qualifications are more vague.

(continued)

EXHIBIT 6.1: JOB POSTING FOR AN ACADEMIC NURSING POSITION (*continued*)

This instructs you to only submit a cover letter and a CV/resume only.

Supplemental Information

Applicants must submit a cover letter, CV/resume; applicants will not be considered until both are submitted.

This statement indicates no formal deadline for submitting an application, although there may be a date when they would like to fill the position.

Review of applications will begin immediately and continue until the position is filled.

For more information, email Geri Havemore, PhD, RN,

SON, Search and Screen Committee Chair

at havemore@BobU.edu.

The contact person is the chair of the search committee, NOT the dean, department chair, or the university's human resources department. They will accept the initial application materials by email.

If you are invited for an interview you will need to provide **official** transcripts and three professional references

If contacted, you will be asked to present official transcripts of your highest degree earned at the time of interview and the contact information of three professional references.

ALL MATERIALS MUST BE ATTACHED WHEN SUBMITTING THE APPLICATION. THEY CANNOT BE REVISED OR ADDED ONCE THE APPLICATION HAS BEEN SUBMITTED.

Once you submit materials you can't revise them.

Step 3: Write the Application Letter

Once you have (honestly) determined that you meet the qualifications and have some expertise in performing the duties of the position, your next step is to write the application letter. To assist you in writing this letter you need to have the two preliminary documents that were previously described in this chapter: the table matching your expertise and experiences with the duties and responsibilities of the position, and the table listing the unit's goals and how you can contribute to these goals. A written application letter for an academic position serves a number of purposes for your potential employer as exhibited in Exhibit 6.2. First, this letter illustrates your ability to follow directions and to express yourself through a written medium. Since writing is the medium by which scholarship is communicated in academic nursing, your application letter will indicate to your prospective employer your potential to be a productive scholar. Second, your application letter informs your potential employer how you meet or exceed the qualifications of the position and how by hiring you the institution will move toward its goals. A common error job seekers make in their application letter is they describe their professional goals and how the institutional resources can help them achieve those goals. Instead, the applicant needs to emphasize how their qualifications and experiences can contribute to the institution's goals. If you are asked to describe your professional goals, they need to be consistent with the goals of the institution and thus, both you and the institution are working toward the same thing. The third and most important purpose of your application letter is to persuade your potential employer to invite you to the next step in the hiring process, which is an interview. Clearly state that your qualifications and experiences have prepared you to successfully engage in the roles and responsibilities of the position to meet the institution's strategic goals.

EXHIBIT 6.2: SAMPLE APPLICATION LETTER

(The contact person listed in job posting.)

Geri Havemore, PhD, RN
Search and Screen Committee Chair
School of Nursing, College of Health and Human Services
Bob University

Dear Dr. Havemore,

I am applying for a 10-month tenure-track faculty position ~~beginning in fall [year]~~ at the School of Nursing at Bob University. I believe I am uniquely qualified for this position as evidenced by my previous

(Key words from the job posting.)

teaching, service, and **contributions to the nursing body of knowledge** in

(Key words from the job posting.)

adult-gerontology. For the past 3 years, **following graduating with my DNP,** I have been an Assistant Professor at Susan University,

(I meet the first requirement of the position.)

College of Nursing. **This position has involved teaching didactic and clinical courses within the second degree and BSN under-**

(Introduce previous experience teaching, serving on committees, and participating on interdisciplinary projects)

graduate nursing programs, serving on numerous school and university committees, and participating on interdisciplinary projects. Also, while working at Susan University for the past 3 years, I have remained

(I meet the second requirement of the position.)

current with my clinical skills by maintaining a clinical practice as a nurse practitioner at the Barrio Guadalupe Family Clinic. Prior to this appointment, I was completing my DNP program in nursing at Melinda University and the title of my capstone project was "**An Evaluation of Teaching Breast Feeding to New Mothers Using Virtual Reality.**" As evidenced by my previous employment and

(Provides some insight into content expertise in the area of family health/obstetrics.)

professional activities, I believe am a viable candidate for the position of Assistant Professor within the School of Nursing at Bob University.

(continued)

EXHIBIT 6.2: SAMPLE APPLICATION LETTER (*continued*)

Introductory sentence explains that this paragraph will contain information about teaching, service, and knowledge-building activities.

Since being appointed at Susan University 3 years ago I have engaged in a variety of teaching, service, and knowledge-building activities. I began by participating as a member of the team of faculty teaching NUR344 Family Health Nursing. As part of this team, I developed lectures and simulation experiences to teach anatomy and physiology and nursing assessment skills of new mothers and newborns. I went on to lead this team of faculty for the past 2 years in teaching not only NUR344 but also coordinating the clinical experiences of 90 students completing NUR345 Community Health Clinical Nursing. These experiences demonstrate that I have the ability to develop, present, and evaluate content in anatomy and physiology and basic nursing assessment skills. I also acted as the academic advisor for 32 undergraduate nursing students and maintained 10 hours of open office hours per week. Also, during my tenure at Susan University, I served as a member of the search committee for the Associate Dean for Research and as a member of the undergraduate curriculum committee within the School of Nursing. **Finally, I presented the results of my DNP capstone project at the Midwest Nursing Research Society Annual Conference as a scholarly poster presentation and have published the results of this project in the *Journal of Nursing Education.***

Demonstrates the preferred qualification of scholarly productivity.

I believe I am a viable candidate for a 10-month, tenure-track faculty position at the School of Nursing at Bob University because my qualifications and experiences have prepared me to contribute to the number of the strategic goals of the School of Nursing. I am uniquely qualified to contribute to the **university's mission of excellence in teaching** as evidenced by my experiences in developing course content and leading faculty teams teaching in undergraduate nursing programs. Further, I am prepared to contribute to **the School of Nursing's goal of extending knowledge through continuing my program of scholarship** in developing innovate approaches to teach breast feeding. I am committed to preparing caring and competent professionals to enhance health and quality of life within the global community as evidenced by

Explains how the job seeker is qualified to contribute to the university's mission.

Explains how the applicant will contribute to the school's strategic goals.

(*continued*)

> **EXHIBIT 6.2:** SAMPLE APPLICATION LETTER (*continued*)
>
> continuing to supervise students while working at the Barrio Guadalupe Family Clinic.
>
> I would be pleased to schedule a phone interview or campus visit if the search committee believes I am a worthwhile candidate. Thank you for your consideration and I look forward to hearing from you in the future.
>
> Sincerely,

Step 4: The Interview

Based on your application letter and CV, you are invited for an interview. Depending on the position, the interview may involve a number of phases including a telephone/video chat, an airport interview, and/or a campus visit interview. I recall seeing a job posting for a position in Hawaii and thinking that going through the interview process would at least get me free round-trip ticket to Hawaii. After investigating the interview process for this position, I learned there were a series of video chat interviews and required written responses to 10 questions about my vision for the position before I would undergo a same-day airport interview in Denver. The institution would not arrange a campus visit to Hawaii without vetting a pool of serious and qualified candidates. The reason for an interview is to determine if you can contribute to the mission and goals of the institution.

You will need to take a number of preparatory steps before participating in any of these types of interviews. First, sanitize your web presence. Any postings on any social media sites by you or your friends that portray you as anything but a professional, competent scholar need to be removed. For example, that coveted Live2Party@.com email address you created during your undergraduate education needs to be suspended. Those pictures of you at your friend's bachelorette/bachelor party (you know the ones . . .) need to be deleted. Commonly, prospective employers will scan the web for postings that include your name to see "what you are really like." If you would like to find out what is in cyberspace about you, one approach is to Google yourself. During interviews, I have been asked about some of my web postings and struggled with responding to some of the interviewer's questions about my less professional postings. For example, an interviewer once asked me, "I noticed on a social media posting that you are a member of a group named the 'Cat-Splat Society.' I live with three cats. What does your group think of cats?"

The second step in preparing for the interview is to be familiar with everyone who is interviewing you. You should investigate their background, whether you share any common interests, or if there any other common points of curiosity. For everyone you are scheduled to interview with, review his or her online profile on the university's website and review anything they have written lately. You may discover potential collaborators or individuals who control access to key resources or the coach of the soccer team at the school your daughter will attend if you are offered the job. People respond positively to others they believe share their background or interests. People also respond positively if you pay them the compliment of knowing and recognizing their skills and previous achievements. For example, my interviewer became visibly more interested in talking with me during an interview once I mentioned that I had recently read one of his published articles. During another interview, I commented that the interviewer and I shared a work history at the same hospital and probably knew several of the same nursing staff. By mentioning the interviewer's background and interests it demonstrates you have invested time and effort into learning more about your potential coworkers and your commitment to getting the job and being successful.

Also, when preparing for an interview, practice how you will interact with people you will meet. If you have limited experience making presentations, practice your scholarly presentation in front of a mock audience and have them ask you questions they believe the audience may pose during your interview. For example, practice answering the common questions of "What is your future scholarly trajectory and how will you achieve that trajectory at this school?" Try to anticipate possible questions and practice giving aloud your responses including "Why are you interested in this position?"; "What are your professional goals?"; or "Tell me about your strengths and some areas of growth for you." In Table 6.1 you will find examples of strong and weak responses I have encountered to these questions during interviews. In general, the weak responses focus on how the institution can help the job applicant while the strong responses involve how the job applicant can contribute to the institution.

TABLE 6.1 Weak and Strong Responses to Common Interview Questions

Interview Question	Weak Response	Strong Response
Why are you interested in this position?	I have a colleague, Dr. Jill Chillax, who works in the school's simulation laboratory. She told me how great the faculty are to work with here. My nephew also went to school here in engineering and got his degree in 2016. As well, my parents are getting on in years and working for the School would allow to be close to them.	I presented at the Sigma Thea Tau conference last spring and happened to meet a few faculty from your school at the expo area and then later going to their presentations. After talking with the faculty, it seemed like my training and experience in community health could really fit well within your undergraduate program needs and the university's commitment to community participatory research. During the conference I really enjoyed Dr. Lu's presentation on her research regarding parent adherence to a diabetes protocol with their children and can see some similarities between our research. I would love to have her as a mentor.

(continued)

TABLE 6.1 Weak and Strong Responses to Common Interview Questions (*continued*)

Interview Question	Weak Response	Strong Response
What are your professional goals?	Someday I'd really like to try my hand at academic administration. Maybe department chair or research dean (totally unrelated to the college/university). Of course, my plans are to work hard to become an excellent teacher and to continue my research in the area of soybean farmers' health.	My professional goals are similar to the goals that have been outlined in the strategic plan for your school. In particular, the goals of fostering an inclusive learning environment and intensifying the quality and quantity of research and community partnerships within the school of nursing stick out to me. My main goal is to find an even balance with teaching and research that allows me to continue growing in both. In order to meet this goal, I would like to find a faculty mentor who is willing to help me with the nuances of adjusting to a new faculty role and find information about internal and external funding opportunities for research. I'd also like to continue attending and presenting at professional conferences both to continue my own education and to disseminate my work and support from the school to do that would be useful.
Tell me about your strengths and some areas of growth for you?	My strengths are I love to teach and see students grow as a result of what I am teaching them. Some students are harder to reach, but those are the ones I get the most gratification in watching grow and be successful. I also love the scholarly process and developing new knowledge that people can use. One of the challenges I see coming here is finding collaborators to mentor me to sharpen my teaching skills.	I consider one of my biggest strengths to be my affinity for technology. I am quick to learn and adapt to new programs and hardware and to integrate them into my teaching and research. I have found that students appreciate the variety and use of technology beyond PowerPoint. On a similar note, since I'm new to the faculty role, I see this as a major area for growth. Being new, I haven't yet taught a very large variety of courses but this also means that I am not yet set in my ways and very open to feedback and trying new things. I am looking forward to exploring any mentoring opportunities that may be available to improve my teaching skills.

The final preparatory step is to learn as much as you can about the school where you may be working. Learn about how the school strives to achieve its strategic goals. Learn about recent faculty and student accomplishments. You might even figure out where to park your car. Understand the organizational structure of the school, who will be your boss, and who controls the resources you will need to access. Learn about the criteria your interviewers use to evaluate you during your interview. During the interview, most of the individuals you meet with, generally the faculty, can provide feedback about your qualifications and a recommendation about hiring you to the search committee. Exhibit 6.3 is a candidate evaluation form that faculty complete to evaluate a faculty job applicant. Obtaining a copy of this evaluation form prior to your interview may help you emphasize certain content in your responses to questions during your interview. Some unimaginative search committee members even ask their questions directly from the candidate evaluation form. One important document you will need to review prior to your interview is the faculty handbook. This document includes the policies and procedures that guide the day-to-day activities in the school including position descriptions, bylaws or how the organization is governed, and general policies for running the school. The faculty handbook also includes policies for annual reviews and the review process for faculty undergoing reappointment, promotion, and tenure. Pay special attention to this section of the faculty handbook because it includes a description of the process and criteria by which you will be reviewed annually for any merit raises and periodically for promotion. During your annual or periodic review, you will be asked to describe and document how you are meeting or exceeding the criteria for your position and/or rank. For example, if one of these criteria are to "provide evidence of extramural funding of scholarship," you will need to provide this evidence when you undergo any periodic review for position and rank. During your interview you may ask for clarification on any of these criteria. You may also need to refer to this section of the faculty handbook when negotiating if you are offered the position.

EXHIBIT 6.3: CANDIDATE INTERVIEW EVALUATION FORM

Candidate Name: **Job Title:**

Date of Interview: **Interviewer Name:**

Competency	Candidate Rating *	Job Relevancy
Communication: Candidate expresses thoughts clearly in writing and verbally; projects positive manner in all forms of communication; responds diplomatically.	Weak Average Strong	Very Relevant Somewhat Relevant Not Relevant
Problem Solving/Decision-Making: Candidate demonstrates ability to make decisions; involves others as appropriate; demonstrates ability to resolve issues.	Weak Average Strong	Very Relevant Somewhat Relevant Not Relevant
Building Trust: Candidate demonstrates ability to keep commitments and meet deadlines; exhibits integrity and honesty with colleagues and customers; demonstrates ability to be open to views of others; takes responsibility for own actions in a conflict resolution.	Weak Average Strong	Very Relevant Somewhat Relevant Not Relevant

(continued)

EXHIBIT 6.3: CANDIDATE INTERVIEW EVALUATION
FORM (*continued*)

Conflict Resolution: Candidate demonstrates ability to resolve conflict with person directly involved; demonstrates active listening skills; focuses on conflict resolution, not blame.	Weak Average Strong	Very Relevant Somewhat Relevant Not Relevant
Teamwork: Candidate demonstrates ability to work as part of a team; seeks the perspective and expertise of others; looks for opportunities to support others on the team.	Weak Average Strong	Very Relevant Somewhat Relevant Not Relevant
Student/Customer Service Oriented: Candidate demonstrates strong customer service orientation with the ability to provide clear, consistent information and service; demonstrates ability to handle difficult customers; delivers service in a timely and professional way.	Weak Average Strong	Very Relevant Somewhat Relevant Not Relevant
Work Experience Rating: Does candidate possess experience directly related to the position? Weak Average Strong		
Describe candidate's work experience as it relates to the position.		
Job Knowledge, Skills, and Abilities (KSAs) Rating: Weak Average Strong		
Describe candidate's job KSA as it relates to the position.		
Describe candidate's unique skills important for the position/department.		
Overall Assessment: Weak Average Strong		

As you can see from the personal story at the beginning of this chapter, an interview for an academic position can be a day-long or multiple-day process. Just because you have sent the institution your CV and application letter does not mean everyone you meet with during your interview has read these materials. Be prepared to provide information, again, that is included in your CV and/or your application letter. As well, the individuals who interview you will not want to review information already available in the public domain on the university website. Avoid asking questions of your interviewers when the answers to those questions are stated clearly on the institution's website. For example, asking the interviewer if the school has a PhD program when the program is clearly described on the website informs the reviewer that you have not sufficiently investigated the school and you are poorly prepared for the interview.

During the academic interview you will commonly be told the next steps in the process following your interview. This may include when the search committee anticipates completing all their interviews and when they will make a recommendation to the dean about whom to hire. In most schools of nursing, the dean makes the final decision about which candidate to offer a position. Another important fact to keep in mind is your interview does not end until you arrive home. I recall interviewing a highly qualified candidate for an associate dean position who took 10 minutes quizzing the waiter during our dinner, in a very condescending tone, about the gluten content of what seemed like every item on the menu. Although unrelated to this individual's qualifications for the position, this behavior spoke volumes about their interpersonal style. Following the interview, compose a thank-you email to each individual who met with you and mention some component of your conversation. This demonstrates that you value the time they took to meet with you. Also, and equally important, write a thank-you email to all the staff members who assisted in organizing your interview. You may be working with these staff members in the future and you want to leave them with a positive impression because they do control critical resources within the school that you will need to be successful.

Step 5: Negotiation

The negotiation for the position is sometimes the hardest part of the process of securing an academic position. In general, nurses are poor negotiators. The vocation of nursing is based upon caring, empathy, self-sacrifice, and taking care of others sometimes at the nurse's own expense. Although noble, these characteristics that make great nurses do not make great negotiators. During the negotiation process for an academic position, put aside your empathy for the institution and your drive for self-sacrifice for the greater good. When beginning a negotiation there are a few points to keep in mind. First, do NOT begin to negotiate a position before you are offered that position. During an interview you may be asked about resources you might need to be successful if you were offered a position. You may even be asked about resources available in your current position. Be honest in your responses to these questions. The interviewer is trying to determine if the prospective institution has the resources available to include in a possible job offer.

Second, if you receive a job offer, understand that this offer will not be rescinded because you ask for additional resources. Consider the initial job offer as the baseline from which to start negotiating. Job offers rarely decline in available resources being offered during the negotiation process. Third, understand that after you accept a job offer, the negotiation for additional resources as part of the offer is over. The only time to ask for additional resources to be included in a job offer is before you accept the offer. Fourth, make a list of essential resources that you must have to be successful in the position and resources that you would like to have that will make the position more pleasant. On this list include the rationale for how these resources will contribute to your success and ultimately benefit the institution. Describe how these resources will facilitate you meeting or exceeding the criteria for your position, rank, and promotion. Table 6.2 provides an example of essential and preferred resources and an explanation for how these resources will contribute to the strategic goals of the unit, the faculty, and exceeding the criteria for your position, rank, and promotion. Without these rationales the institution or the dean has no incentive to provide these resources and the negotiator will see your request for these resources as self-serving rather than serving the needs of the institution. Notice how the rationales provided in this table include primarily benefits to the institution in the form of providing better academic programs, scholarly productivity, and increased service activities.

TABLE 6.2 List of Negotiated Resources with Rationales

Resource	Rationale
Annual salary of $ XX	This salary is consistent with the 50% percentile for the most recently published data from AACN salaries for Assistant Professors in this region.
Full-time summer teaching appointment for 3 years	In order to increase my teaching experience and deliver high quality didactic content. Being on campus year round will also facilitate my consistent research trajectory and services to the school, university, and the profession.
Consistent teaching assignment of the same courses for the first 3 years	In order to develop, constantly refine, and improve course content and my expertise in delivering the content to students through innovative approaches including service learning experiences, problem-based learning, and use of the simulated or interprofessional learning experiences. This consistentcy in my teaching assignment will also free me from completing in-depth prep for any new courses I am assigned to teach.
Start up research funds of $XX/year for 3 years • External research mentor • External reviews of grant proposals • Editing of manuscripts	These funds will support achievement of publishing at least one data-based manuscript per year, making at least one scholarly presentation per year, and submitting at least one proposal for extramural funding per year.

(continued)

TABLE 6.2 List of Negotiated Resources with Rationales (*continued*)

Resource	Rationale
Access to or purchase of • Eliza Plate reader • Biodex isokinetic dynometer • 70-degree freezer • SPSS, EndNote, Survey Monkey • Laboratory to collect data	Access to these resources are essential to continue my research in the area of health promotion activies on the physiologic functioning of older adults. Without these resources I can not immediately conduct preliminary studies that will provide the foundation for extramural proposal submissions.
Teaching assistant 5 hours/week for every class with enrollments >30 students	The teaching assistant can assist in content delivery and grading exams, which will make time available for further course development, research productivity, and service activities essential to merit promotion and tenure.
Research assistant 10 hours per week for 3 years	The research assistant is essential to conducting small preliminary studies to establish feasibility of the protocol. The RA's contribution will involve coauthoring abstracts and manuscripts and may contribute to their dissertation or research course work.
Individual office with phone, computer with MS Works and Internet connection, desk, computer camera, printer/scanner/fax, window, book shelves, file cabinet	Resources necessary to teach in-class and on-line courses and to maintain research records. An individual office is essential to confidential meetings with students and collecting data from research participants via phone calls/Skype.
Travel $XX/year for 3 years	To make scholarly presentations to meet the criteria for promotion.
Four tickets to two men's basketball games	One of the potential extramural funders of my past and future research is Health Products Inc. My contact at this company is Peter Wannabe who is a fan of college basketball. Attending a few games with him would allow me the opportunity to discuss future funding of my research and how my research may benefit their company.

The first step in the negotiation is usually a phone call from the dean who will make a verbal offer. This verbal offer commonly includes a starting salary, a start date, and any other terms that were discussed during your interview. No matter how favorable the terms of this initial offer are, DO NOT IMMEDIATELY ACCEPT THIS INITIAL OFFER. Through negotiation this offer will only improve and at worst, remain the same. As well, you need to contemplate this initial offer perhaps in consultation with family and friends before making a decision. On one occasion, I simply repeated back the dean's verbal offer and paused for 5 seconds, to which this dean responded, "Well, of course, we can offer you an additional $5,000 because of your experience." If this initial offer does not include everything you need to be successful in the position, inform the dean that you would like some time to consider the offer and that you would like to share the table of resources you developed and the rationale for these resources that you will need to be successful. Sharing this table will allow the dean to understand the reasons for your request and how the institution will benefit by providing you with these resources. At this point in the negotiation, the dean will balance the school's ability to provide these resources with the benefits that would come from providing these resources. Commonly, the dean will "counter" your list of resources with what he or she can and cannot provide. At this point the dean is likely making a final offer and you need to decide if you can be successful at the institution with the resources that are available to you.

CONCLUSION

This chapter described the general process of locating, applying for, interviewing, and negotiating an academic position. The five steps in this process involve creating various written documents. Some of these documents are formal parts of this process (e.g., the application letter) while other documents are to help you clarify your thinking about the position. If you adhere to these steps you will increase your probability of securing an academic position in which you will be happy, successful, and adequately compensated. It is not essential that you complete any of these steps in order to secure an academic position.

REFERENCES

American Association of Colleges of Nursing. (2018). *Nursing faculty shortage*. Retrieved from http://www.aacnnursing.org/News-Information/Fact-Sheets/Nursing-Faculty-Shortage

Boyer, E. L. (1990). *Scholarship reconsidered: Priorities of the professoriate*. Lawrenceville, NJ: Princeton University Press.

Marquette University. (2018). *Marquette University vision statement*. Retrieved from http://www.marquette.edu/about/mission.php

Robertson, F. (2016). Maslow's hierarchy of needs. In M. Wright (Ed.), *Gower handbook of internal communication* (2nd ed., pp. 143–148). New York, NY: Routledge.

The University of Iowa. (2018). *Strategic goals of the college of nursing*. Retrieved from https://nursing.uiowa.edu/about-us/strategic-plan

CHAPTER 7

RESPONDING TO FEEDBACK

Jennifer Avery

"That was excellently observed, say I, when I read a passage in an author where his opinion agrees with mine. When we differ, there I pronounce him to be mistaken."

—Jonathan Swift (Swift, 1887)

PERSONAL STORY

As other chapters have mentioned, no person's writing is the picture of absolute perfection. Nothing has made this more evident or toughened up my skin quite like writing a manuscript based on my dissertation. Advisors, committee members, journal reviewers and editors, fellow students, other nonnursing friends, and family members provided (mostly) invaluable feedback that helped to shape my final dissertation manuscript. Sometimes, it was like a nice pat on the back, the feedback was extremely positive and it felt great! I was on the right track and must be doing an excellent job, this is a breeze! However, just as often, it felt like the feedback was questioning me or incongruent with my opinion, and at times it became challenging to address. I mean, how could I tell someone whose opinion I respect that I disagree with them? In addition, I was also occasionally provided with some less than helpful feedback such as conflicting comments that negated prior ones, or comments about things that were required and could not be changed (e.g., from my husband, "I hate this font," and "Your reference format is stupid" [he really is not a fan of American Psychological Association format]). I avoided, procrastinated, made excuses, and put off responding to all the seemingly negative feedback because it felt like a chore. I thought "Why are *they* doing this *to me*?" I probably spent more time responding to feedback than I did writing the whole dissertation! I needed to change how I approached receiving and addressing feedback, and once I did, the entire process became easier. My reviewers were not "out to get me," they were trying to help me clarify my writing. Without all the feedback and the back and forth responding to it, my writing would have been subpar and, likely, would not have conveyed the message that I intended.

INTRODUCTION

Picasso signed his art so everyone would know who created it. In that way, he invited critique of his work. As an author, you are doing the same. You will find the very process of putting pen to paper invites feedback from a wide variety of sources, whether you requested it or not. Gaining and responding to feedback is an expected "part of the deal" when you tackle projects such as a capstone, a dissertation, or a manuscript for publication. The purpose of this chapter is to provide you with recommendations and resources for responding effectively to that feedback to enhance, rather than stifle, your writing. First, this chapter discusses why you need to seek feedback of your writing and the characteristics of the feedback you may receive. Next, this chapter establishes a plan of attack for addressing criticism and critique of your writing followed by a peek behind the journal editorial curtain with recommendations for responding to journal reviewers and editors. Finally, this chapter provides you with a template for responding to manuscript revisions.

SO. . . DO YOU LIKE IT?

Feedback-seeking is an important part of learning, improving performance, and adapting to new positions or organizations (Crommelinck & Anseel, 2013). Seeking and receiving feedback through mentorships, performance evaluations, and patient surveys is frequently second nature for nurses. Yet, it is easy to shy away from this behavior when it comes to our writing. When you ask for feedback, you expect to be questioned or to receive some suggestions for changing your work (after all, you do not grow by having people tell you things you already believe). What you do not expect, and might even fear, is someone being harsh or personal when providing the critique or telling you something you do not want to hear. Perhaps they suggested you wasted your time in writing your manuscript. Negative feedback such as this can be particularly demoralizing. So why would someone want to subject themselves to that? Why is it essential that we seek feedback on our writing?

The first and most obvious answer is the fallacy of perfection; there is always room for improvement or enhancement or, at least, there is always someone who thinks so. Even published manuscripts or books are not immune. Writing is inherently subjective and open to interpretation. As you seek feedback, you will encounter a plethora of differing opinions in areas such as the word choice, studies you reference, or even the rules of grammar (e.g., the Oxford comma or use of contractions). The challenge will be to determine what among this feedback adds to the quality and/or value of your manuscript versus feedback that goes too far and detracts from your work or is unhelpful. Much like the artist of the Sphinx who chipped away too much and lost the nose, you do not want to chip away at your manuscript and lose the focus of your work. (Side note: There are actually many differing hypotheses related to the missing nose of the Sphinx; however, most of these revolve around environmental wear and tear rather than the over-pursuit of perfection.)

The second and more positive reason for seeking feedback is to gain validation of your work! Feedback allows us to gauge the utility or merit of our product. It reduces uncertainty and lets us know that we are on the right track and that the message we are trying to convey is clear and concise. This feedback also serves as motivation for continued productivity.

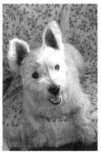

Who's a good boy? Positive feedback works for everyone!

Finally, consider for a moment, what is the end game of seeking feedback. It is to improve your product. You want to put your best foot forward when submitting your work for a grade, grant, conference, or publication. The best way to do so is to seek feedback so you gain an outside perspective of your manuscript before entering the realm of no return (submission). Will it be the end of the world if you do not submit your best work? Highly unlikely, unless your work were to prevent some world-ending disaster. It is more likely that you will not receive the grade, grant, or publication you were pursuing. As such, it is imperative to seek out the right type of feedback and have a set plan for responding to it.

THE WHAT/WHEN/HOW OF FEEDBACK

What is the "right" type of feedback? At what point in the writing process do you need to get feedback? To answer these questions, we first need to talk about the characteristics of feedback. In particular, we will start by focusing on criticism versus critique.

Criticism Versus Critique

Criticism is feedback in which the reviewer/reader takes the "easy way out." Criticism is the identification of problems with a document with no direction about how to fix those problems. Criticism is sometimes termed "constructive," in which the problems are identified in a civil tone, for example, "I don't understand what you're trying to say" or "This section is vague." Destructive criticism is more confrontational

> **WRITING TIP**
> In the words of Ice Cube, "Chickity-check yo self before you wreck yo self."

and may take the form of a personal attack. The following is an example of such an attack: "This section doesn't make any sense. You need to get an editor to clean this up . . . perhaps your 6-year-old" (Bass, 1997). Criticism, whether constructive or destructive, is easy to deliver since the individual delivering the criticism does not have to identify an approach to fixing the problem(s). Unlike criticism, critique is intended to provide the author with direction to improve the document. Good critique provides three levels of detail: (a) what is done well and/or what can be improved, (b) how it can be improved, and (c) why should it be improved. Table 7.1 provides an example text excerpt with both criticism and critique comments directed toward the text.

TABLE 7.1 Feedback Examples

Example Text*	Much is known about the effects of sugar in the diet, but little is known about the effects of a 100% high sugar diet. The purpose of this study is to evaluate the differences of a 100% candy bar vs. 100% ice cream diet among older adults for weight loss. The research question guiding this study was will adults who maintain a consistently unhealthy diet lose weight?	Author Response
Constructive Criticism	"The significance of this study isn't well supported."	
Destructive Criticism	"What is the point of this?" "Were you dropped on your head in grad school?" "Who would fund this study?"	
Critique	"It would be beneficial if you identified the specific type of candy bar and ice cream used in this study. Including this detail would be helpful in being able to replicate the study."	

*Example text created by the author and not representative of an actual study.

When and How?

Now that you know the characteristics of criticism versus critique, the next step is to determine when and how to seek out this feedback. The most obvious (and shortest) method is any time within the writing process from conception to dissemination. The earlier you seek out feed-back on a project, the greater the likelihood that you will identify major problems and prevent little problems from becoming much larger ones later. Seeking feedback is an excellent way of practicing self-reflection and becoming a better writer. One challenge to seeking feedback is that your writing may be still in the formative stage and susceptible to "reframing" or having the message of the document changed by the individual reviewing your document.

There are many ways you can seek feedback, and the main method is peer review. In scholarly writing, peer review involves the process of subjecting your work to the scrutiny of others who are "experts" in the same field. The following two-step process describes how to have your work peer-reviewed.

The first step is to identify the appropriate person(s) to do the re-view. You might need someone with content expertise to critique your research methods, or someone with editorial experience to assess your formatting. You might also seek out feedback from nonnursing profes-sionals to help increase the clarity of your writing through identifying jargon and areas of confusion. Friends and relatives can offer an "out-side" opinion. However, there is a pitfall with this method; friends and family like you and usually want you to succeed so their reviews may be somewhat biased. If you are uncertain about who should review your work, turn to your mentor(s) and peer(s) for advice. You might also consider asking for reviewer-identification advice on an online message board of a professional association or contacting the editor of a journal you want to publish in for their advice.

Once you have identified a good reviewer, step two is to ask for and negotiate the terms of the review. In your request for a review, indicate (a) why you are asking that person to review your work, (b) the scope and purpose of the review that you are requesting, (c) a deadline for when you need the review to be completed, (d) a thank you for the reviewer's time, and of course (e) a copy of the work that is to be reviewed. The deadline is especially important to include, unless you enjoy someone sitting on your work indefinitely. Be considerate of your reviewer's time when requesting feedback on your work. While it may feel tremendously important to you, it may not be a high priority for the reviewer. Unrealistic deadlines, such as a 24-hour turnaround, will not likely be well-received. You must also remember that reviewers are people, too! They can procrastinate, miss deadlines, or may not be as thorough in their review as you would like. As such, consider asking more than one person to review your work to gain multiple perspectives (or at least to ensure you receive one review).

You cannot expect to get peer reviews without giving peer reviews. You will be asked to review another's work. Remember that while it is quick and easy to identify problems via criticism, critique is the more useful and time-intensive form of feedback. Be sure that you identify the positive aspects of the work you review in addition to areas that need improvement. Communication is key when providing critique, so be mindful of your tone in your feedback. In my early peer reviews, I found that my critique was sometimes taken negatively because it was blunt and to the point, which was misinterpreted as cold and uncaring. All the while I thought that I was being concise and clear. However, after hearing those comments and gaining further experience receiving peer reviews, I identified how my communication style inhibited the reception of my critique and then changed how I provided feedback. Do not be afraid to discuss the peer reviews you provide or receive with the reviewee/reviewer as it can provide valuable insight.

PLAN OF ATTACK

You have requested and just been given feedback on your work. Now what? Establishing your plan of attack is a three-step process: (a) prepare your mind, (b) wait and digest, and (c) construct your response. For step one (prepare your mind), make sure you are alone and in the right frame of mind to get a bit verbally beaten. Sit in an oversized recliner with a glass of cocoa, eat some chocolate chip cookies, and snuggle with a teddy bear are some suggestions. Remember, nothing is perfect and if you ask for feedback on how to improve your work, you will get it! There will always be suggested "improvements" or changes to your work and, hopefully, those will be more positive than negative. If a reviewer has a lot of feedback, he or she likely spent a significant amount of time with your work, indicating their commitment to it. Do not worry about the minutiae of the comments in your first reading. Instead, skim the comments to get a general idea of your next steps, and then put it aside; it has been a long day. Right now you may be entering the first stage of Dr. Kübler-Ross's Stages of Grief: shock (Table 7.2; Kübler-Ross & Kessler, 2005). I have unfortunately found myself in shock after a first reading on more than one occasion thinking, "I cannot believe they didn't love it! Did they even read what I wrote??"

TABLE 7.2 Feedback Stages of Grief						
Feedback Action	**Stage of Grief**					
Day 1: Skim Day 4ish: Read a second time	Shock	Denial	Anger			
Day 9ish and beyond: Read a third + time • Share with coauthors • List critique • Make a decision about what you are going to do				Bargaining	Depression	Resolution

Step two (wait and digest) is planning your attack to responding to critique: Wait 2 or 3 days (you heard me right, *days*) and then read the feedback a second time. Time between readings will allow you to bask in the anger and denial stages, which you may have already entered shortly after exiting the shock stage of step one. The anger and denial stages remind me of the frustration that came with reading feedback from a journal reviewer who had obviously not read my manuscript. I was given the comment "no power analysis reported" right below where I reported the [expletive] power analysis in the manuscript (obviously, I am still not over it). The reviewer also said the work was "not significant." Of course the work was significant! Why would I do a study that was not significant? This was the denial talking. I reviewed the same feedback a few days later and I was able to more effectively interpret this comment to mean that I had not explained the significance of the study clearly enough. (Sidebar, instead of a laptop or mobile device, always use a desktop computer to view your feedback or print it out. It is much harder to pitch a desktop against the wall when you read an especially maddening comment. If you print it, then you always have something you can rip up or shut away in a drawer.) Complete step two with a cup of chamomile tea, meditation, and yoga to help take the edge off the anger.

Finally, we come to step three (construct your response) and the real, physical part of moving on to the acceptance stage of grief—responding to the reviewers. This is also a good time to involve your peers to help you dissect the feedback. Yes, this could be a solo activity, but where is the fun in that? Just as your peers can give feedback on your work, they also can help generate ideas on how to translate and respond to the feedback you have received from others. To start dissecting your feedback, you and your peers can evaluate the themes of the reviewer comments. One way of doing this is by using the Feedback Dissection Checklist (Table 7.3).

TABLE 7.3 Feedback Dissection Checklist

Check Off	What Does the Feedback Say?	What Should You Do About It?
☐	No purpose statement, hypotheses, and/or research questions identified.	So why did you write the manuscript? Or was the reviewer blind and missed these elements? Either add the forgotten elements or kindly indicate in your response to the reviewer how/where they are in the manuscript.
☐	No theoretical framework addressed.	Was your framework implied but not stated? Or was there really no framework for your study? Consider how to make your framework or lack thereof (with reasoning) clearer.
☐	Literature cited is too old. *and/or* Seminal works not cited.	If the reviewer suggested particular articles, consider if they fit with your work. Work on citing updated literature or defend/clarify why you are instead citing older studies.

(continued)

TABLE 7.3 Feedback Dissection Checklist (*continued*)

Check Off	What Does the Feedback Say?	What Should You Do About It?
☐	Work is not significant, not important, or in some other way is undervalued.	Resist the temptation to harm your computer. Perhaps your work was reviewed by someone who does not value your specialty? How might you include, reinforce, or otherwise emphasize the significance of your study?
☐	Sample is too small or big. *and/or* Power analysis not included.	Did you cite *a priori* or *post-hoc* power analysis to support your sample size? Why or why not? Defend/clarify your sample size to the reviewer (add analyses/explanations if needed).
☐	Inappropriate data analysis and/or interpretation.	Does the reviewer's comment make sense for what you did? Did you have a statistician help with your project? Did you violate assumptions of normality? Lots of things to consider here, so use your school resources and ask for outside help if needed in formulating your response.
☐	Work has several limitations that limit or invalidate the results.	Do you agree with the reviewer? Did you acknowledge limitations of your work or neglect them? Consider how you can defend the importance of your work despite the identified actual or perceived limitations.
☐	Discussion or conclusions not supported [by data, literature, overall work, etc.].	There are many things that can go wrong in this area. Start by asking once again, do you agree with the reviewer? If you disagree, are you conveying the message that you intend? Again, outside help might be useful in this section to help formulate your response.

Note: The more items you check off, the greater the magnitude of problems with your work. This is not to discourage you but to help indicate how in-depth your revisions may need to be.

The purpose of the Feedback Dissection Checklist is twofold. First, it is there to assist you in dissecting the criticism and critique to identify what the reviewer(s) might have been thinking with their comments. Second, it will help you begin to generate your responses to those comments. Obviously, the fewer items that you check-off on the list, the less editing you will likely need to do. If you find yourself checking off everything, then your manuscript is "perfect," just not in the right direction. Consider using your resources and working with a mentor or writing service to help you dissect the critique. If the feedback was on work submitted for publication or presentation, you may want to consider whether resubmission is appropriate; you may decide that submitting to alternative outlets is a better use of your time.

Creating a Response Table

Once you have completed the checklist, you can translate the identified areas/problems into a response table. If you received comments separate from your manuscript document, like journal reviewer comments, it is helpful to create a table in a separate document presenting the reviewers comments and your response to the comments with the modified text or the specific location of the modified text. This level of detail in your response to reviewers' comments may seem laborious, but it makes the second review of your manuscript much easier for the editor and reviewers. This table easily explains how and where you addressed each of the reviewer's comments. If you adequately addressed each comment, then there likely will be no new concerns to address and your manuscript will most likely be accepted for publication (Table 7.4). If you received the comments within your manuscript (e.g., comments within a Word document), you could either follow the previous suggestion, or you could insert your responses as comments next to the reviewer's comments within your manuscript (see the excerpt from one of my dissertation drafts in Figure 7.1).

TABLE 7.4 Example Feedback Response Table Templates

Response Table 1			
Manuscript Section	**Reviewer Comment**	**Author Response***	**Action Taken**
Line 85	No power analysis reported	Power analysis is reported on line 84	No action taken
No section given	This work is not significant	This study is significant for the following reasons . . . Perhaps these reasons were not well conveyed in the manuscript so additional details have been added.	Revised the background and significance section as well as the study implications section to further emphasize the significance of this study.

Response Table 2	
Concern/Comment	**Revisions/Clarifications***
No power analysis reported	The power analysis in this study was reported just above line 85 on line 84, as such no revisions were made.
This work is not significant.	This study is significant for the following reasons . . . Perhaps these reasons were not well conveyed in the manuscript so additional details have been added. Revisions have been made to the background and significance sections as well as the study implications sections to further emphasize the significance of this study. Changes are highlighted in yellow in the resubmitted manuscript.

*Author responses are abridged.
Note: Consider why you might want to use Table 1 versus Table 2. You will likely use Table 1 the most as it is more specific and contains more detail than Table 2. However, Table 2 is simple and useful when revisions are fairly minor and/or there are few comments to address.

When responding, there are a few key things to remember:

Include unedited comments. Always include the reviewer's unedited comments. Do not delete or ignore a comment just because you do not like or agree with it (as tempting as that may be). You do not have to agree with the reviewer comments, but you do have to respond to *all* of them. Your response may be that you incorporated the recommended changes

Incidence and prevalence of MCI. One recent large-scale ($n = 1944$) study (Katz et al., 2011), using widely accepted criteria (Artero, Petersen, Touchon, & Ritchie, 2006), found MCI incidence rates of 3.8 and 3.9/100 person-years and prevalence of 11.6% and 9.9% for aMCI and naMCI respectively.[LA1] Comparatively, in the same study, for all types of dementia the incidence rate was 2.9/100 person-years and prevalence was 6.5% (Katz et al., 2011). Katz et al. (2011) also noted higher rates of naMCI in persons who identified as African American/Black compared to Caucasian/White. African American/Black race was also found to be a significant risk factor for development of MCI in the Cardiovascular Health Study (Lopez et al., 2003). Other studies have found conflicting results, with incidence rates of MCI among Hispanic/Latino and African American/Black persons similar to the incidence rates of MCI among Caucasian/White persons (Manly et al., 2008; Unverzagt et al., 2011). These conflicting results suggest that the differences of MCI incidence by race may be contributed to increased misclassification of MCI (Kennedy, 2011). In general, it has been estimated that MCI affects approximately up to one in five older adults globally (Laino, 2011).

The general rate of progression from those diagnosed with either subset of MCI to dementia is estimated to be around 10% per year (Petersen, 2011). However, the speed of progression (i.e. months versus years) from MCI to dementia is inconsistent and difficult to predict (Portet et al., 2006). In addition, there is little evidence to suggest which potential factors might influence or lead to one MCI subset over another, or which factors might influence a person's transition/speed from MCI to dementia (Alzheimer's Association, 2011). The higher incidence and prevalence of MCI versus dementia, and the potential progressive relationship between MCI and dementia highlights the possibility of a large portion of adults progressing from MCI to dementia in the not so distant future. [LA2] It suggests a need for increased primary care..

> **Local Admin**
> Think about rephrasing to put incidence rates at beginning of sentence for greater impact
> Ok, moved beginning sentence to end of paragraph to begin paragraph with this

> **Local Admin**
> Can these be combined for greater succinctness?
> Ok, deleted "extremely concerning and beginning of next sentence to combine them

FIGURE 7.1 Dissertation draft excerpt. Reviewer comments were made by the "Local Admin," then my responses are highlighted. This is an actual example from one of the many drafts of my dissertation.

or that you chose not to make the change. If you choose not to make suggested changes or address a comment, then you need to explain why you made this decision. "Because I said so," or just "no" are not appropriate justifications. Quite often, revised submissions are critiqued by the original reviewer, and these comments will not go away during the next review. Also, by not addressing a comment, you run the risk of appearing not to value the reviewer's feedback, and your resubmission may not be considered. You may also receive conflicting comments when you have multiple reviewers, but this does not mean you can select the one you like and move on. It likely means that section of the manuscript was not clear. You should acknowledge the conflict among reviewers and explain (as in the next steps) how you have increased the clarity of your manuscript.

Provide rationale. You must provide some supported rationale for each response. In Figure 7.1, I created a scenario that is a good example of what not to do because I did not provide rationale for the edits.

Instead, I only provided some indication of agreement and a description of what I changed (however, I was also meeting one-on-one with the reviewer to discuss the rationale). If you only tell the reviewers what you changed and not why, it can be interpreted as you making edits without clear purpose. In other words, you made changes to the manuscript just because the reviewers suggested those changes. You must always be purposeful (e.g., provide increased clarity, address specific review questions, fix errors), and not merely revise the wording in the hopes that the reviewers will think you addressed their concern.

Identify change. In your response, let the reviewer know if you changed content. You may have deleted statements or added references or, if you rejected the suggested changes, state your rationale for not making the suggested changes. As seen in Table 7.4, you can include an "action" column to make your revisions obvious to the reviewer. Keep in mind that just because a reviewer comments on something, that does not mean you are *required* to change it. It is perfectly acceptable not to act on a comment if you can provide adequate justification for why you chose not to act. The more obvious and straightforward you can be with your response/action the better. Using this method also gives the reviewers a clear idea if their comments were misinterpreted. It also gives you a history of what changes a reviewer suggested so you have something to reference if that reviewer provides conflicting feedback in a later draft. In general, if you receive conflicting feedback, whether it be from the same person between drafts or from two different reviewers on the same draft, it is a good indication that something is confusing or ambiguous about that section or statement. Either provide more clarity or ask yourself if that information is essential to the manuscript. If it is not, delete it.

BEHIND THE CURTAIN

Now that we have discussed the types of feedback and how to effectively respond to that feedback, it is time to take a peek behind the journal editorial curtain. We begin with the reviewers who put the "peer" in peer review. Who becomes a journal reviewer? That all depends on the journal. First, if you have submitted a manuscript to that journal, then you may one day be asked to review for it. The first manuscript that I coauthored during my graduate program was the product of a project with the dental school. It was published in *Gerodontology* (an international journal pertaining to oral health and older adults). Shortly after the manuscript was submitted, I received an invitation to review two manuscripts for the journal. My first thought was, "I'm not a dentist," followed by "I'm just a student, why are they asking me to do this?" and ending with "Why in the world do they think I am qualified to do this? I have had cavities!" I did eventually review at least one manuscript for the journal, as it was within my scope of practice and was something about which I had knowledge, or perhaps expertise. If you are competent enough to write for a journal, then you may also be asked to review for that journal.

Second, instead of asking authors to review, the journal may request peer reviews from their review board. The review board is different from an editorial board. Review boards are generally volunteer positions and selected through both self and peer nomination. Nominations usually involve sending in a copy of your CV with description of why you want to be a reviewer to a journal editor who then approves and selects the new board members. The terms of being a board member vary by journal and are usually 1 to 5 year commitments.

Third, many journals are associated with different professional organizations. As such, members of those professional organizations may receive requests to serve as reviewers for their respective journals. You may also meet journal editors within your professional organization(s) who may ask you to serve as a reviewer for their journal(s). In one study, the most frequently listed reason for being a peer review at 24% ($n=349$) was contact with an editor through means such as peer networking, meeting at a professional event, or email correspondence after submitting an article to their journal (Kearney, Baggs, Broome, Dougherty, & Freda, 2008). Finally, when you submit a scholarly manuscript for peer review, you may be asked to provide a list of names of other professionals who might have the expertise to review your work. You may have colleagues ask if they can list you as a potential reviewer for their work, but I would suggest that you read Chapter 9, Difficult Documents, before you agree to this.

Now, you may be thinking at this point, "Okay. That explains the reviewers, but what about the editors?" Similar to newspaper publishing, the number and source of editors depends on the size and scope of the journal. Many editors are often involved in a hierarchical function and their level of contribution to the journal may vary. Titles and roles of different editors vary across journals and may include in no particular order: editor, editor-in-chief, executive editor, associate editor, assistant editor, senior editor, managing editor, editorial board member, contributing editor, and copy editor. The point is, editor roles vary and there may be more than one editor in contact with you at each stage of the submission process. Editor positions are often part time, secondary to academic or other positions, with salaries ranging anywhere from $0 to $80,000 per year (averaging $13,000-$39,000 per year), depending on the journal type (scholarly vs. magazine) and number of submissions (Freda & Kearney, 2007). These positions are sometimes term limited with upward of a 5-year term length, and those terms may or may not be renewable (Freda & Kearney, 2005). Editors (regardless of type) are the gatekeepers of their journals. They decide which manuscripts will be peer reviewed and, ultimately, which manuscripts to publish. They also set journal policies, write contributing columns, solicit for submissions and reviewers, and are responsible for upholding the overall quality of the journal (Freda & Kearney, 2005).

NO . . . NO! . . . OR NO WAY EVER?

Now that you know who is involved with peer-reviewed journals, we can talk about the review process and the types of decisions. When you first submit your manuscript, an editor receives it and decides to either reject the manuscript without further review (usually within the first week of submission) or send it on for peer review. If at this point your manuscript is returned to you with not undergoing peer review (NO!), do not despair! Instead, consider the editor's comments (if any constructive suggestions are provided) and either resubmit (if comments indicated that a resubmission would be entertained) or submit your manuscript to the next journal. Sometimes it can be difficult to dissect an editor's comments. For example, you may be told that your manuscript is "not suitable at this time." Which could mean that your manuscript would be suitable at that journal in the future (No?), or it could just be that editor's way of letting you down softly, "It's not you, it's me" (No way ever). You can wait and resubmit your manuscript in the future, or you can submit to another journal.

Once your manuscript goes on to peer review, the process can take around 4 to 6 weeks (or whatever time frame the journal has published). If after 3 months you have not heard anything from the journal beyond confirmation of your submission, try calling or sending a follow-up email asking for the status of your manuscript. If you do not get a response to your follow-up or that response is unsatisfactory, then you may wish to withdraw your manuscript from consideration in that journal. Finally, if all goes as planned, the peer reviewers send their feedback to the journal editor with their recommendations and comments, then the journal editor will make the final decision regarding publication. This process is illustrated by the decision tree in Figure 7.2.

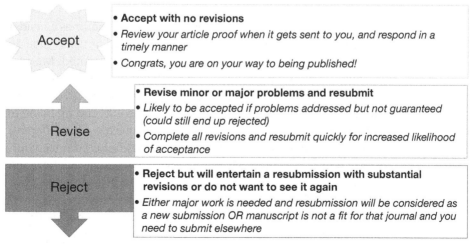

FIGURE 7.2 Editorial decision tree.

While you may think that you have the perfect manuscript, there is a high probability that no one else will, except for a pet goat. Only 8% of papers "win the lottery" and are accepted on their first submission without revisions (Freda & Kearney, 2005). It is more likely that you will be asked to make revisions based on the peer review feedback and then resubmit. The letter that you receive may even appear like a form letter, similar to one parodied by Dr. Jorge Cham of PHD Comics (http://phdcomics.com/comics.php?f=1888). Unfortunately, editorial feedback is not always as clear as simply asking you to make revisions; the feedback may even be masked in jargon. In Table 7.5, I have translated some common editorial phrases.

TABLE 7.5 Editor Translator

What the Editor Said	What the Editor Means
Please address the reviewer comments and resubmit your work by 10/10.	I have an issue in mind for your work, you had better complete the minor revisions and resubmit on time for me to publish it.
We regret to inform you that your manuscript has been rejected due to major concerns. However, if you wish to address these concerns we would welcome your resubmission.	Your manuscript is in need of major revisions, but I am still interested in it. So please consider revising it and sending it back!
Your manuscript is not suitable at this time (and/ or needs substantial revisions), but please consider resubmitting.	Your manuscript likely needs major work but may still be of interest to the journal if we release a call for manuscripts and it fits the theme.
Your manuscript is not suitable at this time and if you decide to resubmit please contact me before doing so. OR Your manuscript is not suitable at this time for this journal.	Either your manuscript is in need of major work or really just wasn't a fit for the journal (e.g., submitting a manuscript focused on geriatrics to a pediatric journal).
Your manuscript is not suitable for this journal.	I do not expect you to send this in again; please do not bug me about it.

Being asked to complete minor revisions is sometimes considered as "conditional acceptance" in that the changes are not extensive and the review process on the resubmission is often abbreviated. Make sure to complete any minor revisions and resubmit as soon as possible while your article is of interest to the journal. You will be given a due date, and if you wait too long, your resubmission could end up being treated as an entirely new submission. Major revisions are a bit different; even if you complete those major revisions, it does not guarantee your manuscript will be accepted. Major revisions also take more effort and time to complete but still should be completed as soon as possible and before the due date. Upon resubmission, the same peer reviewers may review your manuscript if they are available, or your work may go through an entirely new review process. Differences between some common minor versus major revisions are illustrated in Table 7.6.

TABLE 7.6 Differences Between Minor and Major Revisions	
Minor Revisions	**Major Revisions**
• Editing	• Narrow the purpose
• Additional literature	• Revise statistics
• Revise background or discussion	• Add or change theoretical framework
• Format changes	• Collect more data
• Clarify methods	• Major rewrite to align background, methods, results, and discussion
• Shorten or lengthen	
Source: Courtesy of Robert Topp.	

Your Editorial Decision

> **WRITING TIP**
> For every manuscript there is a journal waiting to publish it!

At this point you now have a decision to make. You can (a) revise and resubmit, (b) revise and submit to a new journal, (c) submit to a new journal without revisions, (d) protest/appeal the decision. Remember, if less than 10% of papers are accepted on their first submission that means that more than 90% are rejected in one form or another and necessitate resubmission. For option (d), there is little benefit to protesting or appealing an editor's decision (for further detail, see Chapter 9, Difficult Documents), and generally, you would still need to complete revisions before your manuscript is ready for publication. Option (c) can be a viable path but only if your manuscript was rejected because it did not fit with the journal and if little or no feedback was provided. Your best options are (a) and (b).

When you revise and resubmit to a journal, you need to include a response letter and the edited manuscript in addition to any other files requested by the editor. In your response letter, first thank the editor and peer reviewers for their consideration and the opportunity to revise, and for their comments, time, and effort. Next, acknowledge the revisions that you have made in your manuscript and indicate that you have included a response table following your letter (always include a response table like the example in Table 7.4). Finally, end your letter by once again thanking the editor and reviewers for considering your resubmission and how their feedback has strengthened the quality of the paper. See Appendix 7.1 for an example template for this letter.

When you revise and submit to a new journal, you do not need to include information about the previous journal that you submitted to, feedback that you received, or a response to the reviewer comment table. However, it is almost always a wise idea to revise your manuscript based on the peer review feedback you have already received. You can then submit your newly revised manuscript to the next journal. It is possible that the journal, even upon rejection, may leave open the possibility for a new submission once major changes have been made to the paper. It may warrant a brief contact with the editorial team to determine if this is an option, especially if you are convinced their journal is the best fit to reach your intended audience.

CONCLUSION

Have you made it through the Stages of Grief intact? The purpose of this chapter was to provide you with recommendations and resources for responding effectively to feedback that will enhance rather than stifle your writing. This was accomplished through first discussing reasons for seeking feedback on your writing and identifying types of feedback, including differences between criticism and critique. I then laid out a plan of attack and gave you a feedback dissection checklist to help you interpret and respond to your feedback. Finally, this chapter ended with a brief peek behind the editorial curtain and a letter template for responding to editors.

REFERENCES

Bass, B. M. (1997). Does the transactional–transformational leadership paradigm transcend organizational and national boundaries? *American Psychologist, 52*(2), 130–139. doi:10.1037/0003-066X.52.2.130

Crommelinck, M., & Anseel, F. (2013). Understanding and encouraging feedback-seeking behaviour: A literature review. *Medical Education, 47*(3), 232–241. doi:10.1111/medu.12075

Freda, M. C., & Kearney, M. (2005). An international survey of nurse editors' roles and practices. *Journal of Nursing Scholarship, 37*(1), 87–94. doi:10.1111/j.1547-5069.2005.00006.x

Freda, M. C., & Kearney, M. H. (2007). A first look at nurse editors' compensation. *Nursing Economic$, 25*(6), 371–375.

Kearney, M. H., Baggs, J. G., Broome, M. E., Dougherty, M. C., & Freda, M. C. (2008). Experience, time investment, and motivators of nursing journal peer reviewers. *Journal of Nursing Scholarship, 40*(4), 395–400. doi:10.1111/j.1547-5069.2008.00255.x

Kübler-Ross, E., & Kessler, D. (2005). *On grief and grieving*. New York, NY: Scribner.

Swift, J. (1887). Thoughts on various subjects. In R. Cochrane (Ed.), *The English essayists: A comprehensive selection from the works of the great essayists from Lord Bacon to John Ruskin with introduction, biographical notices, and critical notes*. Edinburgh, UK: W. P. Nimmo, Hay, & Mitchell.

APPENDIX 7.1 RESPONSE LETTER TEMPLATE

Potat Ohead, PhD, WHNP-BC, RN
Senior Editor, Journal of Nursing and Cat Toys

Dear Dr. Ohead,

> Step 1: Thank the reviewers for their consideration of your original submission, their comments, time, and effort.

Thank you to you and the reviewers for your consideration and thoughtful comments regarding my manuscript, *A Phenomenological Inquiry of Why Weebles Wobble But Do Not Provide Good Pain Control*. I greatly appreciate your time and effort in providing me with feedback. This manuscript is being resubmitted only to the *Journal of Nursing and Children's Toys* (JNCT) for consideration for publication.

> Step 2: Tell the Editor what you did. Acknowledge the revisions that you have made and indicate that you have attached a response table a la Table 7.4.

Based on your recommendations, I have made a **number of revisions** to the manuscript and I am hopeful that my revisions will address the concerns that were raised. Please see the attached "Response Table," which explains my revisions and responses to the reviewer comments. In addition, all changes are highlighted in yellow in the manuscript.

> You could also say that you have made "minor" or "major" revisions that were requested

Thank you for entertaining my resubmission. My manuscript explored the lived experience of those attempting to use Weebles for pain control and identifies several areas for consideration in nursing practice. As the *JNCT*'s mission is to publish articles that advance the science of children's toys in nursing practice with an emphasis on qualitative studies, I believe that my manuscript will be of interest to the journal reviewers and readers. I look forward to hearing your decision regarding publication. Should you have questions about my resubmission or need further information, please contact me via the details below. Thank you.

> Step 3: Thank the editor and reviewers again for entertaining your resubmission and indicate your hopefulness for publication in the journal. Making sure to indicate the fit of your manuscript to the journal mission/theme is helpful, too.

Sincerely,

Barrel 'Om Onkeys, PhD, CNE, RN
Assistant Professor
Bob University, Timbuktu
Office: 123-456-7890
Email: bonkeys@bob.edu

CHAPTER 8

TEAM WRITING: PLAYING WELL WITH OTHERS

David Vance and Joseph Perazzo

PERSONAL STORY

I decided to go back to graduate school because I was lucky to have met a lot of amazing nurses who pursued careers in research and wanted to do the amazing work that they did. While I was a graduate student, I got involved with a team of researchers in my field for some hands-on experience. I knew they did not have any money to pay me, but I also knew the professional growth I would gain would make it all worthwhile. I dove into the experience, becoming involved with every aspect I could. I transcribed the lead scientist's handwritten notes and turned it into a functioning protocol that we submitted to the institutional review board for ethics approval. I spent much of my free time in hospital waiting rooms to recruit participants for the study and obtained informed consent from potential candidates. I collected data, entered the information into the data management system, and cleaned it so it was ready to analyze. Once we had collected all the data, I took part in weekly meetings to review the results. It had, by this time, been over a year since I had started. One of the study team members asked me if I would like to "take a stab" at writing the background and methods sections for a manuscript the team would submit to a scientific journal. He did not have to ask me twice. I wrote my draft, ran it by a good writer I knew, made some suggested revisions, and sent it to the team. I got an email from one of the team members thanking me and telling me that they would be in touch.

A few months later, the entire team received an email from the lead investigator with a subject heading that read "Way to go, team!" I scrolled down to see that our manuscript was accepted for publication!

I accessed the article through the school library and opened it. There it was! My writing in a published article! There was just one problem. While my writing was there, my name was not. I was not an author. I was not even in the microscopic font that acknowledges study team members. I emailed the lead scientist to see what we could do to fix this mistake. His reaction surprised me to say the least. He wrote, "Your efforts are certainly appreciated. I think the best thing to do is keep jumping in where you can, and down the road, we can talk about authorship on publications. I'm sure you would agree you are getting great experience working with us!" It knocked the wind out of me. It felt wrong and unfair and I was not in any hurry to "jump in" on any of their projects. However, he was right in that it was a good experience. After all, I have never made the same mistake again.

INTRODUCTION

Nurses are members of highly skilled teams across settings, from the bedside to the classroom. Whether it is working on a class assignment, a dissertation, a DNP project, a conference presentation, or a manuscript for a journal, nurses often find themselves writing in teams. The experience I shared may seem extreme, but it is a story I hear all the time, particularly from students assigned to work on a project as a group. Who is in charge and who is the straggler? Whose idea is best? And of course, who should get credit for what? I admit that there have been many times when working on a team that I have wanted to take the reins and just get a project done rather than worry about someone else's schedule. I like feeling in control of my work and my timeline. However, that does not mean that working alone is always the best idea. I am one person with one experience. My knowledge base is limited to my experiences, and as a researcher, my work often reflects the collaborative effort of individuals from multiple professions. This chapter is dedicated to writing as part of a team. In this chapter, I will discuss the benefits and challenges of writing as part of a team, provide some tips on optimizing the experience of writing on a team, and present a few helpful templates you can use when you are writing on a team.

THE BENEFITS OF TEAM WRITING

Networking

Whether you are working in the hospital setting or in academia, submitting projects to journals and conferences is important and can be a great way to network with others (Holzemer, 2007). For example, if you are on a unit that has implemented a change in patient care, you can partner with fellow nurses and other healthcare workers to disseminate your project. Many long-term professional collaborations and friendships begin in exactly this way. Joining together with others for a common goal is a great way to find common ground that is mutually beneficial.

Expertise

No one person knows everything (I know, I was shocked when I found out, too). There are times when writing alone is expected, such as writing a paper in a specific course, a dissertation, or a capstone paper. Authors may also fly solo when writing commentaries, editorials, blogs, novels, or focused writing in their area of expertise. However, in the case of scholarly writing (e.g., to report on research projects or academic programs), authors often blend and compile expertise (Street, Rogers, Israel, & Braunack-Mayer, 2010; Vance, 2014). They may be in different professions or areas of a shared profession. They may have different training and, thus, provide an entirely different perspective on a given topic. While it can sometimes be hard to play well with others, this sort of team work helps people overcome individual limitations. Working with a diverse team of experts often leads to opportunities you may have not thought of yourself. For example, team members may suggest journals and conferences you were not familiar with but those suggestions will expand your work in scope and reach an entirely unexpected audience outside of nursing. It is important to embrace the contributions of people who have different expertise. It is equally important to share what we know as nurses outside of our discipline.

Sharing the Workload

As you have read throughout this book, the entire process of writing includes more than typing words on a computer. It includes all the activities that generated something to write about, including conceptualization, background research, the activities of a project, compiling literature, identifying a journal (in the case of publication), and then, of course, putting those words on paper. It can be an overwhelming prospect for one person to do everything alone. Working as a team helps to "share the wealth," reducing individual workload and thereby decreasing the amount of time it takes to complete a project. In addition to splitting up the overall process, the writing itself can also be split up into sections, which can help bring the final work together quickly (Vance, 2013, 2014).

Increased Quality

Something that happens to me when I have been working on a writing project for an extended period is that I almost do not see my own errors anymore. A major benefit to partnering with others is the work is seen by multiple sets of eyes. We are all human and when we are our only critic, anything from a grammatical nuance to an outright error in logic or fact can go unnoticed. Working with others almost always improves the quality of the work because they can help provide initial critique and integrity to the work (Vance, 2013, 2014). In the end, team work pays off! Whether it is finishing an assignment or project, or receiving the notification that you are to be published, it is a great feeling to have accomplished something together as a team (Figure 8.1).

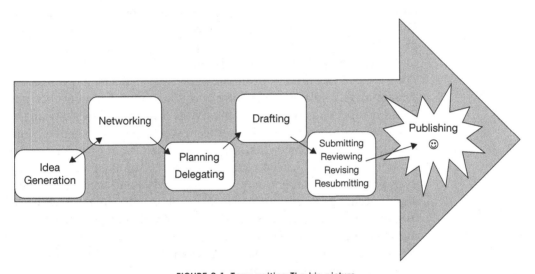

FIGURE 8.1 Team writing: The big picture.

CHALLENGES TO TEAM WRITING

Authorship

As described in Chapter 2, Why Do We (Have to) Write?, authorship is the currency, or the bread and butter, of academics. It is the way that academicians show what they have been doing with their time and is a major deciding factor for reappointment, promotion, and tenure (Resnick, 2015; Street et al., 2010; Vasconcelos, Vasgird, Ichikawa, & Plemmons, 2014). While it may seem at first that arguments over authorship order are petty ego battles, there is often a deeper issue. New scholars frequently have difficulty with this topic because they receive many opinions. Scholars have had many lengthy debates about who should be awarded authorship and in what order they should appear on a paper. Some believe that unless you have been responsible for actually writing part of the paper, you should not receive authorship and instead should receive an acknowledgment. Meanwhile, an equally fervent group of scholars will tell you that involvement in a project should award an individual authorship regardless of involvement in writing the manuscript. When the issue of authorship is not clearly described prior to developing a manuscript, it can cause a lot of hard feelings and professional rifts. It is always a good idea to consult nationally recognized guidelines on this topic while making these decisions.

Managing the Moving Parts

When you get a group of busy people together to work on a project, it can be like herding cats to get the final product together. A reality to collaborating with others is that the brainstorming phase (e.g., ideas for a project or paper) is often full of lofty promises and big ideas. When there is no structure in place and everything is left open-ended, it can be a maddening task to keep everyone on track. One gets very used to hearing the phrase, "I have just been so busy. . .". Fortunately, in the next section we offer some solutions to this very common problem.

Broken Continuity

One challenge when writing as part of a team (primarily when the actual writing is divided among team members) is you may deal with a disjointed piece of writing. A reader will be able to easily see there were many hands involved because the paper does not read well (Vance, 2014). This can be particularly frustrating when you are up against a deadline. However, as you will read in the next section of this chapter, you will find this is a relatively easy fix.

Disagreement

Varying points of view are a good thing. They provide challenges to your way of thinking that truly can strengthen your writing. The flipside is that disagreements can create a bottleneck in the writing process when people with opposing views dig in their heels. It is common for these disagreements to have more to do with conflicting opinions and preferences and less to do with conflicting science.

STRATEGIES AND SOLUTIONS

While team writing does come with potential challenges, they are not prerequisite to working on a team. There is a growing body of strategic wisdom on the subject because enough people have had (and continue to have) these experiences. In the next sections, I present you with some strategies you can use to promote the benefits and prevent the challenges.

Consult Experienced Authors, Journals, and Professional Organizations

Experienced authors, journals, and professional organizations have long understood some of the complications that come with team publishing (see the references at the end of this chapter). Consulting these resources can help you learn about important factors to consider when determining the writing workload and the order of authorship among team members. While there are variations, there are some notable consistencies across these resources:

- Who holds intellectual property rights for the work? (e.g., Who conceptualized the project? Whose research question guided the efforts? To whom do the data belong?)

- What was the involvement of the team member in the project? Did they conceptualize, do the footwork, help write the paper, or all of the above?

- No one should be "gifted" authorship! Being an author suggests involvement in the project/analysis/write-up. It is important to note that just as there are nurses who do not wash their hands, there are people who engage in giving authorship to people who have done nothing on the project—it does not mean it *should* happen! It is quite literally something that your name is on, so you want to make sure it is done with integrity.

- All authors should agree upon workload, authorship, and the final product. No one author should do most of the work for nothing or very little work for everything.

Step up as a Leader

When collaborating with others, I have noticed that people sometimes avoid structure and leadership so they do not appear to be controlling or tyrants. However, stepping up as a leader is invaluable to the team even though it is something many people would rather not do. For example, people may need reminders or encouragement during the project. It is easier for one person to compile and track different documents or versions of the manuscript. A major role of the leader would be to help finalize the manuscript. A manuscript that has been written by many hands can appear disjointed due to language variation and writing skill. If you are the first author (or an experienced author on the team), it is always a good idea to do a careful editorial review of the final draft of the manuscript. Revisit the paper for consistent terminology, verb tenses, and voice (e.g., ensuring first and third person are in agreement). Where applicable, minor changes can be made to promote consistency and structure to the manuscript. Remember, the best manuscripts are the ones that are easy to read! It can be intimidating to assume a leadership role, but if you follow through, it is an invaluable contribution to the team writing process.

Do Not Wing It—Make a Plan and Put It in Writing

Planning is a crucial component of successful team writing. Structure will be your best friend, as it will put all the team members on the same page. This piece of advice applies to so many aspects of life, and team writing is one of them! While there are times that projects evolve (e.g., new team members come on board or drop off, new data are added), writing a paper is not a difficult task to plan. Once you decide to write something, contact your team with a proposal. Include a proposed workload for the paper, the authors you will include (with justification, if appropriate) in the order they will be listed, and solicit agreement or feedback. Set a deadline for contributions as necessary and a proposed date of submission to the journal. Make sure you are also up-front with guidelines so you are not bogged down with minutiae at the last minute. As your team may include inexperienced writers, discuss the tense in which the piece will be written (past vs. present), limits on the number of references and cut-off dates (e.g., no older than 5 years from the time you are writing).

A well-laid plan, while not always perfect, gives team members the opportunity to provide feedback while documenting a solid plan to move forward. It also prevents the disasters that can accompany word-of-mouth or inconsistent agreements among the team. If something changes, inform the entire team and obtain agreement again. See Appendix 8.1 for a template of an authorship agreement that you can modify and use at the beginning of a writing project.

Be Accountable and Expect Accountability

A great way to avoid misunderstandings and keep the team on track is to set up a plan for accountability. I cannot count the number of times I have been in a situation when working with a group when I have said, "I have not heard from so-and-so for a while. I wonder how they are progressing on their section of the paper." After waiting an appropriate amount of time to ask (so I do not sound like I am harassing), I have often heard, "I am sorry, I haven't even had time to look at that. Things have been so crazy." I have had much better luck working with teams when there is some form of regular meeting or check-in on the project. In addition to promoting accountability, you continually renew opportunities for people to share ideas, insights, or even the difficulties they are having with their workload. Accountability does not always mean that you "do it now and do it right." It could mean that a person is simply unable to hold up his or her end of the deal and some revisions to the workload need to be made.

Respect the Team and Yourself!

Last (but certainly not least), it is crucial that team members work together in a spirit of true collaboration. Every team member should leave the experience feeling as though they benefited from their participation. People run into complications when there is a lack of respect for others, whether it be their effort, their time, or their position. It is important to note that with varying backgrounds and perspectives come misunderstandings. Someone may appear to be careless with a deadline when in fact they are overwhelmed. Conversely, no one should expect you to put your own work on hold because they were not communicative. Every situation is different, but if you apply some of the strategies described in this chapter, you can avoid unnecessary tension or discomfort among team members.

CONCLUSION

In this chapter, you have learned about the benefits and challenges of writing with a team and some strategies you can use when writing with a group of people. The personal story I shared at the beginning of the chapter is a case study that underscores the need for this chapter. I do not believe that anyone set out to upset me. I was working on a team that had very conflicting ideas on what was required for authorship, very little planning or defining of responsibility, and poor communication among team members. The result reflected those dynamics. I learned a lot from the experience and if I can help you avoid the same mistakes, it was time well spent. Now go, team!

REFERENCES

Holzemer, W. L. (2007). University of California, San Francisco international nursing network for HIV/AIDS research. *International Nursing Review, 54*(3), 234–242. doi: 10.1111/j.1466-7657.2007.00571.x

Resnick, B. (2015). Academic authorship guidelines for capstone and dissertation work. *Geriatric Nursing, 36*(6), 421–422. doi: 10.1016/j.gerinurse.2015.10.001

Street, J. M., Rogers, W. A., Israel, M., & Braunack-Mayer, A. J. (2010). Credit where credit is due? Regulation, research integrity and the attribution of authorship in the health sciences. *Social Science and Medicine, 70*(9), 1458–1465. doi: 10.1016/j.socscimed.2010.01.013

Vance, D. E. (2013). To write alone or not to write alone, that is the question. *Nursing: Research and Reviews, 3*, 43–46.

Vance, D. E. (2014, May-June). Solo vs collaborative scientific writing models: Balancing the advantages and disadvantages. *Research Practitioner, 15*, 59–64.

Vasconcelos, S., Vasgird, D., Ichikawa, I., & Plemmons, D. (2014). Authorship guidelines and actual practice: Are they harmonized in different research systems? *Journal of Microbiology and Biology Education, 15*(2), 155.doi: 10.1128/jmbe.v15i2.867

APPENDIX 8.1 AUTHORSHIP AGREEMENT DOCUMENT

PROPOSED PAPER

Secondary analysis of Dr. Mentor's caretaker survey data. Dr. Postdoc completed a secondary analysis looking at testing the relationships between mental health diagnoses and caregiver role strain from data collected in Protocol ABC-12345.

Start your authorship agreement with a statement of the purpose; in this case a plan to submit a secondary analysis to a journal.

STUDY TEAM MEMBERS

Be transparent about authorship; in this case, three of the five study team members will be authors on the paper.

Team Member	Responsibilities	Authorship?
Dr. Mentor	Principal investigator of protocol	Yes
Dr. Postdoc	Co-Investigator; leader of present analysis	Yes
Dr. Stats	Statistical support in original protocol and	Yes
John Assistant	Original protocol	No
Jane Associate	Regulatory representative	No

PROPOSED AUTHORSHIP/RESPONSIBILITY

A simple table like this one outlines the responsibilities of each author, but also acknowledges the efforts of the other team members; be sure to compile all funding sources that covered the effort/expenses associated with the study.

Team Member	Authorship/Responsibilities
Dr. Postdoc	**First Author** • Background • Methods • Results (narrative) • Discussion • Correspondence; submission
Dr. Stats	**Second Author** • Results (statistics; tables) • Critical review of final draft • Approval of final draft
Dr. Mentor	**Third (Last/Senior) Author** • Conceptualization • Critical review of final paper • Approval of final draft
Acknowledgments by Name	John Assistant, Jane Associate
Other Acknowledgments	Caretaker Resource Center John Doe Association Funding (Grant 123456789) Jane Doe Research Center Funding (Grant 987654321)

JOURNAL SUBMISSION:

Part of the publication plan should include where you want to submit the paper; give several options in case it is not reviewed or is not accepted at a specific journal.

First Choice: *Family Health*

Second Choice: *Advances in Caregiving*

Third Choice: *Psychology and Disease*

PROPOSED DATES: *

Set your expectations for deadlines and submission dates.

Draft to Team: 12/01/2020

Revisions to Dr. Postdoc: 12/15/2020

Final Draft to Team: 12/20/2020

Submission to Journal: 01/01/2021

*Dates may change if major revisions suggested; new dates to be sent to team if applicable.

By **signing** you agree to the information provided about this submission. Please provide any questions and feedback in writing by [DATE]. If you are at a distance please type in your name and the date along with a written note of agreement and submit by email.

If you work closely with team members, obtain their signature for agreement to the plan for publication; this example shows that confirmation by email is also acceptable in this case.

Team Member Signature _____ Date _____
Team Member Signature _____ Date _____
Team Member Signature _____ Date _____

CHAPTER 9

DIFFICULT DOCUMENTS

Robert Topp

PERSONAL STORY

I have known "Terry" for over 10 years. Her husband, Tom, and I have worked together on projects for national professional organizations and have met socially many times with our respective spouses during scientific conferences. Terry is a faculty member at an academic health center. Terry, Tom, my wife "Schmoochie," and I have talked, over libations, about the challenges of doing human subjects research. We discovered we have all experienced similar headaches with the institutional review boards, with non- or over-compliant subjects, and with getting funded. We have even gone as far as fantasizing about opening "Bob University" where we could proactively solve all the barriers to becoming famous researchers.

Terry emailed me one day and asked if I would be able to provide an external review of her application for promotion. I felt comfortable and competent in being able to provide an unbiased review of her application because we had never collaborated professionally, but I was familiar with the content of her research. A few weeks later the dean of Terry's college sent me an email formally requesting me to provide an external review of Terry's application for promotion to professor. I responded to the dean that I would be happy to provide a review of Terry's application. The following week a 2-inch thick manila envelope marked "Confidential" arrived in my university mailbox. This envelope contained a letter from the dean requesting I submit my written review of Terry's application by a deadline which was 2 months in the future. The letter also instructed me not to contact the candidate, Terry, prior to submitting my review. "No problem," I thought, and without looking at the remaining contents, I placed the envelope on the far corner of my desk with a mental note to look at the packet when I had free time. Five-and-half weeks later on a Friday afternoon, I reopened the envelope and discovered it contained the university's criteria for promotion and tenure, Terry's CV dated 3 years previously, Terry's two-page application for promotion, two complete journals each of which included a single manuscript listing Terry as second and third author, respectively. Also in the envelope were two complete conference proceedings each of which included a single abstract with Terry as the first author. Finally, the envelope contained numerous meeting minutes from school and university committees over the previous 3 years that included Terry on the attendance list.

I read over the university's criteria for tenure and promotion, which included "publishing and presenting an independent trajectory of national and internationally recognized research . . . evidence of teaching innovations and excellence in teaching . . . leadership on university and professional organizations." I started to feel a little sick to my stomach. The "evidence" provided by Terry's application did not match the university's criteria and I was starting to think I was going to be the person to deny Terry's application for promotion and lose my friendship with Tom. This external review of Terry's application for promotion to professor was turning into a very difficult document for me to write! (The conclusion of this story is at the end of the chapter.)

INTRODUCTION

This story is ripe with opportunities for me dodge writing a "difficult document." A difficult document is a document that causes you anxiety when writing it or thinking about writing it. This chapter focuses on difficult documents that involve writing an evaluation of someone else's work product, performance, or productivity and then writing a recommendation about the degree to which the work meets some criteria. Whenever you provide an evaluation and recommendation of someone else's work, the potential exists that your interpretation is not congruent with their opinion of their work and your recommendation could be viewed as bad news or even confrontational. The best way to reduce the anxiety associated with writing a difficult document is to avoid getting into the position of writing the difficult document in the first place. I begin this chapter by discussing behaviors that commonly contribute to the undesirable experience of writing a difficult document. These behaviors include procrastination and not "looking before you leap" into agreeing to write a recommendation for someone. Of course, sometimes there are situations in which there is just no way to avoid the necessity of writing a difficult document. Following this exploration of behaviors that contribute to getting into the position of being unable to avoid writing a difficult document, I will describe the process and content of writing several different types of difficult documents. I will also provide templates for these documents including recommendation letters for an academic position, recommendation for tenure and promotion, recommendation for merit based upon annual review, and grievance or decision appeal letters.

BEHAVIORS LEADING TO WRITING DIFFICULT DOCUMENTS

> **WRITING TIP**
> *If you're going through hell why would you want to stop? Keep going!*
> —Adapted from Winston Churchill

No one wakes up in the morning and thinks "This is going to be a great day because I get to write a difficult document." Writing or sometimes just thinking about writing a difficult document commonly causes the author anxiety. There are two behaviors that contribute to getting into the undesirable position of writing a difficult document. I am guilty of both behaviors, which include procrastination and not fully exploring what writing a recommendation for someone may involve. I also refer to this second behavior as "not looking before you leap" into agreeing to write a recommendation for someone. Procrastination is defined as "the act of needlessly delaying a task to the point of experiencing subjective discomfort" (Solomon & Rothblum, 1984). Many individuals employ procrastination as a coping mechanism to avoid the anxiety associated with writing or thinking about writing a difficult document. I am continually amazed at the effort some people invest in avoiding completion or even starting a task and the mental anguish they endure instead of just doing the work. Robert Peck (2003) was one of the first to recognize the negative effects procrastination can have on enjoying life. To paraphrase this author:

> Life inevitably includes pleasant and unpleasant tasks. We commonly dwell on, obsess over, complain about, feel guilty, and generally try to avoid completing the unpleasant tasks, while pleasant tasks we eagerly complete quickly. This pattern of behavior of procrastinating over unpleasant tasks and quickly completing pleasant tasks results in us spending a greater proportion of our time thinking about or doing unpleasant tasks while spending relatively little time on pleasant tasks.

Figure 9.1 presents pie charts depicting the amount of time people who are high and low procrastinators spend engaged in pleasant and unpleasant tasks. As this figure indicates, those engaged in less procrastination about unpleasant activities will complete these activities more quickly, which allows them more time to indulge in pleasant activities. Those who procrastinate about unpleasant activities will spend more time completing these activities and, in turn, will compound the perception that the activity is unpleasant and requires excessive time to

High Procrastinator

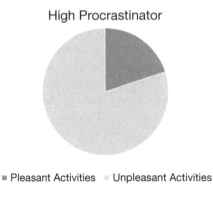

■ Pleasant Activities   ▪ Unpleasant Activities

Low Procastinator

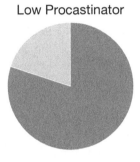

■ Pleasant Activities   ▪ Unpleasant Activities

FIGURE 9.1 Time spent in pleasant and unpleasant activities by low and high procrastinators.

complete. Procrastinating over a difficult document increases the time required to compose the document, which in turn begins a cycle of increasing procrastination, leading to increased time required to complete the document, leading to increased anxiety, leading to increased procrastination in an attempt to mitigate the anxiety, all of which perpetuates the cycle of increasing discomfort and not completing the task of writing the document. Procrastination can contribute to the undesirable experience of writing a difficult document. Constantly thinking about, complaining about, feel guilty about not working on, and generally trying to avoid completing a difficult document commonly results in not completing the document in a timely manner and working at the last minute with the quality of the document being diminished.

The other behavior that may lead you to the undesirable position of writing a difficult document is not fully exploring the request to write a recommendation or evaluation before agreeing to do it or "not looking before you leap into agreeing to write a recommendation." As an academic or professional nurse, you may be asked to write recommendations or evaluations in the form of professional endorsement letters, letters of support for projects, and performance evaluation letters. These requests commonly come from friends, former students, or associates with whom you have a positive personal and/or working relationship.

Additionally, there are times you may be asked to write a recommendation or evaluation for someone you do not know or perhaps someone with whom you do not have a positive relationship. For example, as supervisor, you may be asked to provide an evaluation of a subordinate, or, as a faculty, you may be asked to provide a recommendation as part of a peer review process. You may also be asked to provide a recommendation or evaluation for someone you do not know because of your expertise in a particular field. A recommendation or evaluation may be for a friend or associate, someone with whom you do not have a positive relationship, or for someone you have never met. For all three of these groups of individuals, strive to resist the temptation of allowing your personal feelings for the individual to influence your recommendation or evaluation. If you are unable to separate your personal feelings for the person from your recommendation or evaluation of the person's work product, performance, or productivity, then you will *not* provide an objective recommendation or evaluation. If you cannot provide an unbiased evaluation or recommendation, then simply say to the person making the request, "I do not believe I can provide you with an unbiased evaluation of your work. I want you to be successful in your pursuit of this goal, so I do not want to introduce the appearance of my recommendation prejudicing the process."

Before agreeing to provide a recommendation, you need to "look before you leap" and explore how much work is involved and the nature of the work involved in fulfilling the request. There are two areas you need to explore before responding to a request to write a recommendation or evaluation. First, understand why the individual is seeking you to provide the recommendation or evaluation. Are they seeking your recommendation because of your content expertise, because they are required to because of your professional relationship with the person, because of your familiarity with his or her work, because of your personal relationship with the individual, or because of some combination of these reasons? Understand that if an individual is seeking your recommendation because of your personal relationship, your relationship may suffer if you provide a less than stellar recommendation although secure friendships can endure professional differences. Agreeing to assist friends by providing them with a recommendation or evaluation needs to include clear boundaries between friendship and professional integrity. Without going all "utilitarian" (de Lazari-Radek & Singer, 2017) on you, if you are asked to provide an evaluation of someone else's work product, performance, or productivity understand that you are being asked to provide an objective interpretation or an interpretation that any other person would reasonably provide *based on the evidence* Resist the temptation to offer an unfounded glowing evaluation of your friend's work. As well, fight the urge, as seductive and well-deserved as it may be, to offer an unwarranted damaging evaluation of someone's work when you do not like that person. Evaluations without evidence that are overly optimistic or pessimistic are frequently revealed as biased; once this is revealed, the desired effect of the recommendation will be limited or the recommendation will be disregarded all together. An unfounded recommendation, either positive or negative, will likely damage your reputation to a greater degree than achieving the desired effect, positive or negative, of your recommendation.

> **WRITING TIP**
> Everyone knows that no one likes going into the unknown without knowing.

The second area you need to explore before agreeing to write an evaluation or recommendation is to understand what the process of providing the evaluation involves. What materials are you being asked to review, what are (if any) the criteria that you are being asked to measure the materials against, how much of your time will the process require, and what level of anonymity is provided in the process? This information about the process of conducting the evaluation and providing a recommendation will give you an idea of how challenging the process may be and how much of your time the process may require. Finally, if permissible, you need to have some idea of the level of recommendation you will likely provide and communicate this to the individual requesting your recommendation prior to providing the official written recommendation. This final area may involve completing a preliminary review of the materials about which you are being asked to provide a recommendation. This preliminary review will give you some idea of the level of enthusiasm you will be able to provide in your recommendation. You may wish, if the process permits, to share this level of enthusiasm or your anticipated recommendation with the person asking for your recommendation in case they want to withdraw the request. Be honest and tell them "based on my review of the evidence that you have shared with me, I can provide you with an [outstanding, good, average, or substandard] recommendation." Being honest in telling someone requesting your recommendation your level of enthusiasm for their work prior to agreeing to provide a recommendation will allow the individual to consider withdrawing the request. This preliminary review needs to be completed as soon as the request is made but prior to you committing to providing a recommendation. Completing these areas prior to deciding to provide a recommendation will reduce the number of difficult documents you will need to compose.

PROCESS AND CONTENT OF A DIFFICULT DOCUMENT

There are a variety of difficult documents that involve conducting an evaluation of someone's work product, performance, or productivity and providing a written recommendation about the degree to which the work meets some criteria. The process of preparing these different types of difficult documents adheres to a similar method. First, determine the criteria and then the degree to which the individual's work product, performance, or productivity aligns with the criteria. Sometimes these criteria are objectively quantified as with a grading metric for a class assignment. For example, "students must demonstrate competency with the material by scoring above 78% on a multiple-choice exam." Other criteria are less quantifiable and may require some interpretation by you, the reviewer. For example, criteria for promotion to the rank of associate professor may be stated as "evidence of a sustained program of nationally recognized research." This example requires the reviewer to define the terms "sustained program" and "nationally recognized research." The reviewer may define a "sustained program" as "the individual being principal investigator on studies receiving uninterrupted extramural funding from a federal agency for the past 5 years" or "the individual making a data-based presentation at a national research conference for at least 4 of the 5 previous years." The first step in evaluating someone's work product, performance, or productivity is to determine the objective criteria to which the person's work product, performance, or productivity will be compared. The more objective these criteria are, the less opportunity for interpretation and bias entering into the evaluation and the easier time you will have in developing the difficult document. Commonly what makes a difficult document challenging to compose is the vague nature or lack of criteria on which to base your recommendation of the individual's work product, performance, or productivity. The process of composing a difficult document is first to establish the objective criteria and then to determine the degree to which the individual's work product, performance, or productivity aligns with the criteria on which the person is being evaluated. If the individual's work product, performance, or productivity meets or exceeds the criteria, then you have justification based on evidence in providing a positive recommendation. On the other hand, if the individual's work product, performance, or productivity falls short of the criteria, then a negative recommendation is warranted based on evidence.

The content of many difficult documents adheres to the same general format (see Appendices 9.1, 9.2, and 9.3). The document commonly includes five sections. First, tell the reader the purpose of the document which provides a general introduction to the document. In this initial section, describe why you are writing the document, citing who approached you to write the document, and the nature of the request. For example, you might begin a difficult document with the sentence "I am responding to the request of Dr. Rocky J. Squirrel to provide a professional recommendation as a component of his application for the position of Associate Professor at Whatsamatta University."

In the second section of the difficult document, describe any relationship you may have with the individual you are evaluating and for whom you are providing the recommendation. This disclosure frames your credibility to provide an unbiased recommendation. Describing your relationship with the individual allows the reader to evaluate any potential bias you may covertly or overtly harbor in your evaluation and recommendation. For instance, if you have collaborated daily with an individual for over 20 years by conducting research projects and co-authoring manuscripts, then your recommendation is likely to be positive because of your close working relationship. If, on the other hand, you simply share a common content expertise with the individual to whom you are providing the recommendation, then you are less likely to be viewed as having a working or personal relationship influence your recommendation.

> **WRITING TIP**
> *Try not. Do. . . or do not. There is no try.*
> —Yoda

The third section of the difficult document includes your evaluation of whether the individual's work product, performance, or productivity meets or does not meet the criteria on which the person is being evaluated. In this section, you state the criteria and then present evidence to support if the individual has achieved the criteria. If the criteria are objectively stated and the evidence is clearly provided, then there is limited opportunity for bias or variability in interpreting whether the criteria have or have not been met. For example, "Dr. Squirrel has a sustained program of nationally recognized research as evidenced by publishing four data-based manuscripts as first author and co-authored an additional three manuscripts over the previous 5 years." Another example of how to compose this section when evidence does not match the criteria might be "Dr. Squirrel has been an active member in school and university committees but has not presented evidence that he has volunteered or been elected to a leadership position on school or university committees." In both examples, you are simply stating whether or not evidence exists that an individual's work product, performance, or productivity aligns with the criteria on which they are being evaluated. This third section commonly includes an evaluation of a variety of criteria and whether evidence exists indicating the individual's work product, performance, or productivity meets or does not meet the criteria. Since multiple criteria may be evaluated, it is possible that you may conclude some criteria as being met and other criteria as not being met. Resist the temptation of using ambiguous adverbs or terms in your evaluation, such as "approached the criteria" or "working toward the criteria." Using these indefinite terms does not help the reader in judging whether the criteria were or were not met.

The fourth section of the difficult document is optional. If you are able, provide a description of the individual's interpersonal style along with evidence to support your description. This section provides the reader with your interpretation of how the individual interacts with others. In this section, you are answering the question "Does he or she play nice with others in the sandbox?" Or "Will he or she 'fit' on our team?" This section provides the reader with information beyond the criteria on which the individual is being evaluated and may provide the reader with some insight into the individual's personal strengths and limitations. Again, the interpretation you provide in this section needs to be supported by evidence or examples detailing the individual's strengths and/or limitations. For example, writing, "Dr. Squirrel exhibits several personal strengths that prepare him for a successful career as an Associate Professor at WU. These strengths include promptly returning phone calls and emails, a willingness to contribute to team projects including always attending team meetings, and completing assignments by the predetermined deadlines." In comparison, a less than positive description of an individual's limitations may be stated as, "Dr. Squirrel exhibits a number of opportunities for growth including more promptly returning phone calls and emails, regularly attending meetings, being a more active contributor in team meetings, and being more compliant with predetermined deadlines."

The final section of a difficult document is where you provide a conclusion to the question of whether the evidence aligns with the criteria, and based on that conclusion, you state a clear level of enthusiasm for your recommendation. This final section explains to the reader how you achieved the purpose of the document that you presented in the first section of the document. In this section, provide a clear response to the initial request for a recommendation. Like many nurses, you may want to "comfort the blow" of delivering a substandard recommendation by being vague or evasive in your recommendation statement. Demonstrating concern for others and how your recommendation may affect someone professionally or personally is consistent with our profession's core values (Fagermoen, 1997). However, if your recommendation is ambiguous or noncommittal, the reader will find your document insufficient and you as the author will have failed to provide the recommendation that you said you would provide. If you have clearly documented in section three of the difficult document evidence of how the criteria were or were not met then writing an overall recommendation will be justified. An approach I have found more supportive when delivering a poor recommendation is to provide the recommendation surrounded by positive statements. For example, you might write, "Dr. Squirrel has presented evidence of being well liked by students in his class. Unfortunately, Dr. Squirrel does not present adequate evidence the he meets the criteria for promotion to the position of Associate Professor although his service to the school through chairing the faculty affairs committee for the past 2 years is commendable." Surrounding your recommendation with positive statements may be a way for you to communicate caring about the person you are reviewing while not allowing these positive statements to distract you from your commitment to provide an unbiased assessment of the individual's work product, performance, or productivity.

THE EASIEST WAY TO WRITE DIFFICULT DOCUMENTS

As with most disagreeable tasks in academe that most people do not want to do, if you become proficient at writing difficult documents then you will be asked to do this task more often. As word gets out that you can write a difficult document well, more students, colleagues, and administrators will approach you to provide an evaluation and recommendation of their or someone else's work product, performance, or productivity. You can respond to this increasing number of requests by "cherry picking" to write only the difficult documents that do not consume an excess amount of your time or threaten your mental stability. Commonly, difficult documents that are easy to write are for someone who exceeds the clearly stated criteria on which they are being evaluated. Giving good news is always easier and much more gratifying than giving bad news. Of course, this "slacking" approach will leave composing the difficult document to someone else and others will quickly catch on to your method, causing your credibility to diminish.

A second approach I use when an individual asks me to write a recommendation on their behalf is to ask the requester to provide a first draft of the letter they would like me to write. When using this approach, I will provide the requestor with a template from which to write since most people have difficulty writing about their work product, performance, or productivity (see Appendices 9.1 through 9.4). The template informs the requestor of the five sections of the recommendation and how the recommendation is based upon whether their work product, performance, or productivity meets or does not meet the criteria on which he or she is being evaluated. This approach has several advantages. First, this approach allows you some insight into what the person making the request would like you to say. Second, this approach initially relieves you from identifying the criteria on which the requestor is being evaluated and you avoid the task of initially matching the individual's work product, performance, or productivity with that criteria. Finally, this approach relieves you from sitting down and writing the initial version of the document and, as has been mentioned previously in this text, it is much easier to revise a scholarly document than to create one. Once the requestor gives me the draft of the letter he or she would like me to write, I then rewrite the letter as necessary in order to provide an unbiased evaluation of the degree to which the requestor's work product, performance, or productivity aligns with some criteria and, ultimately, the recommendation based upon that evaluation.

There have been times this approach of having the requestor compose the first draft of the letter he or she would like me to write did not work or "bombed." When this approach fails, it commonly leaves me with more work and potentially compromises my credibility and my personal/professional relationship with the requestor. To avoid problems with this approach, tell the requestor how much time you will

> **WRITING TIP**
> Your collaborator's lack of planning does not constitute your emergency.

need to revise the letter and if you use this approach, give the requestor a deadline for receiving the first draft. Also, tell the requestor that if he or she fails to meet the deadline, you will be unable to provide a recommendation by any deadline the requestor may have communicated. Many people have the habit of working up against a deadline; providing the requestor with a deadline keeps you from having to compose your final version at the last minute. Another challenge when using this approach is when the requestor provides an overly positive recommendation not supported by his or her work product, performance, or productivity. In this case I will inform the requestor that, based on the evidence, I cannot provide the same level of enthusiasm in my final version. I will also tell the requestor that I would be happy to agree with the level of enthusiasm if he or she can provide me with evidence of the work product, performance or productivity that would warrant a higher level of my enthusiasm. Finally, I will inform the requestor of the level of recommendation I can provide based on the evidence provided. This interaction may result in the requestor withdrawing the request for my recommendation or agreeing with my interpretation of the degree to which his or her work product, performance, or productivity aligns with the criteria. Converse to the individual who writes an overly optimistic letter, is the requestor who either minimizes his or her work product, performance, or productivity or "hurries through" the first draft with the expectation that I will revise the letter, aligning the requestor's work product, performance, or productivity with the criteria. I respond to these individuals by saying asking "Are you sure you want me to provide this level of recommendation? Based upon your work product, performance, or productivity, I believe *you* could write for *me* a much more enthusiastic first draft letter." This interaction frequently sends the requestor back to the computer to write a better first draft. On occasion, meek or overly busy individuals will ask me to use the information in the initial letter for my final draft. In this case, the final version of my recommendation is at the level of enthusiasm the individual wants me to advocate.

THE MOST CHALLENGING DIFFICULT DOCUMENTS

The most challenging type of difficult document to write is a grievance or appeal letter. An appeal letter is defined as a letter giving reasons why someone should reconsider a decision they have made previously because you think the original decision was erroneous. Similarly, a grievance letter is a document that provides grounds for a complaint. For the purposes of composing this type of difficult document, the terms "grievance" and "appeal" will be used interchangeably. Most academic settings have a formal process for pursuing a grievance or appealing an evaluation and recommendation. It is critical that you follow the process described by your institution because if you do not, your appeal will not be considered or, worse, you may develop a reputation as someone who does not follow the rules. This will provide evidence that the initial evaluation and recommendation was accurate. As well, if the institutional appeal process involves someone different than the individual who completed the initial review, you may want to keep the initial reviewer informed of your intentions. The rationale for this transparency is so the initial reviewer does not perceive you as subverting their credibility, being deceitful, or being secretive; this demonstrates that you are following the institutional process and respectfully appealing their initial evaluation and recommendation. Keeping everyone involved informed of your intent to appeal the initial evaluation and recommendation and explaining your reasons for the appeal show respect for your reviewers and demonstrate your ability to follow rules.

The essence of a grievance or appeal letter is that you disagree with someone else's interpretation of the merits of your work product, performance, or productivity or the degree to which the evidence meets the criteria by which you are being evaluated. Writing this document commonly occurs when the criteria and/or the work product, performance, or productivity are incompletely presented or vaguely stated. **The objective of an appeal document is to convince the reader to reconsider the initial evaluation and recommendation of your work product, performance, or productivity.** Reconsidering the initial evaluation and recommendation is the first step toward the reader changing the initial evaluation and recommendation, hopefully, for your benefit. Persuading someone to reconsider and revise his or her evaluation and recommendation is a serious challenge because you are trying to convince the reader that the initial evaluation and recommendation were inaccurate—and *no one likes to be told he or she made a mistake or did not do a good job*. So, when writing an appeal letter, there are a few points that you need to keep in mind if you hope to achieve the goal of that letter. First, clearly identify, for yourself, what result you would like from writing the appeal and consider the probability of realizing that result. If your desired result is to publicize the incompetence of the person who provided the initial evaluation and have the person reprimanded and or fired, recognize that this desired result is inconsistent with the objective of an appeal letter mentioned earlier in bold letters. Also, if you think it is unlikely that your appeal letter will convince the reader to reconsider the initial evaluation and recommendation, then writing the appeal may be an exercise in futility for you and irritating for others, which, again, is *not* the objective of an appeal letter. Similarly, do not include personal attacks or other statements the reader could interpret as inflammatory. Remember, the goal of this letter is to convince the reader to reconsider his or her initial evaluation and recommendation. Taking an aggressive position or attacking someone else's abilities will not move you toward this goal. Finally, avoid discussing the work product, performance, or productivity of others in comparison to the evaluation and recommendation of your work product, performance, or productivity. Evaluation and recommendations in academia are overwhelmingly based on objective criteria and not on comparisons among individuals. For example, most promotion and tenure criteria are not stated relative to other faculty's productivity but rather based on objective criteria. As well, grades assigned in academic courses are rarely given based on the other student's work product, performance, or productivity. Mentioning any perceived or actual inconsistencies in the evaluation and recommendation of your work compared to others will likely be considered an attack on the competency of the initial reviewer and counterproductive to the goal of the appeal letter.

The format of an appeal letter is slightly different from the format of the other difficult documents examined in this chapter. First, in an appeal letter, describe to the reader the purpose of the letter, which is to ask the reader to reconsider the initial evaluation and recommendation. Immediately following this request, provide the reader with the rationale for why you believe he or she might reconsider the initial evaluation and recommendation. This rationale is not intended to point out an error in the initial evaluation and recommendation; rather, it should provide the reader with some new information or an alternative interpretation that would justify reconsidering the initial evaluation and recommendation. Commonly this rationale includes additional evidence or an alternative interpretation about your work product, performance, or productivity or clarification of the criteria on which you are being evaluated. If you do not offer the reviewer anything new to consider, then why would you expect them to arrive at a different evaluation and recommendation?

The third section includes content from the original evaluation and recommendation on which you agree with the reviewer's initial account. Come on now, be honest here. If you received less than an outstanding evaluation and recommendation, perhaps there are some areas for improvement or at least some kernel of truth in the reviewer's initial evaluation and recommendation. Acknowledging points of agreement with the initial evaluation and recommendation is important because it indicates "common ground" and content with which you both agree. Similar to responding to critique in Chapter 7, Responding to Feedback, you may even compliment the reviewer's abilities in this section as a way of showing them you do not disagree with their entire assessment and that you appreciate their efforts. Remember, the reviewer had to write the initial evaluation and recommendation, which was likely a difficult document to compose. Following the points of agreement, provide the reader with the *new* evidence that you hope will persuade the reader to reconsider the initial evaluation and recommendation. Again, avoid being confrontational by presenting this new information as previously being overlooked. Do not suggest the initial review was in error or did not attend to details. Rather, present the evidence as new and possibly not available when the reader provided the initial evaluation and recommendation. Remember, the objective of this appeal letter is to convince the reader to reconsider the initial evaluation and recommendation of your work product, performance, or productivity, which is the first step toward he or she changing the initial evaluation and recommendation, hopefully, for your benefit. Thus, in the final section of an appeal letter ask the reader, based on the new evidence, if he or she would reconsider the initial evaluation and recommendation.

CONCLUSION

Difficult documents are hard to write. This chapter has described two behaviors that can ease the agony when writing a difficult document. First, try to avoid procrastinating over writing a difficult document. The longer you procrastinate the difficult the task of writing, the longer it will take to complete the task, and the less time you will be able to pursue more pleasant activities. Also, "look before you leap" into agreeing to write a difficult document. Ensure you understand how much work will be involved and the level of enthusiasm you can provide in your recommendation. Also, ensure the person requesting your evaluation still wants you to provide your recommendation once he or she knows the level of your enthusiasm. This chapter also described the content and process of creating various types of difficult documents including a grievance or appeal letter.

And Now the Rest of the Story . . ..

Recall, at the beginning of the chapter, my story about the "evidence" provided by Terry's application and how it did not match the university's criteria for promotion to professor. I was going to recommend denying Terry's application for promotion and possibly lose my friendship with Tom and Terry. After kicking myself for procrastinating over starting this difficult document and not "looking before I leaped" into agreeing to provide this external review, I began to write. While composing my evaluation and recommendation, I thought about how much Terry complained about always being busy writing articles, preparing new courses, and being an active member of her university senate. I thought "she has some nerve complaining more than I did when in fact it appeared she wasn't doing much work at all." In fact, I was surprised she thought she had the qualifications to even apply for full professor. I was also surprised that her dean even let her apply for promotion when she obviously did not meet the criteria. Then it occurred to me that maybe

Terry was working as hard as she said and maybe the dean was supporting a qualified candidate and that I had not received all of Terry's materials. I called Terry's dean and said, "I do not understand. From what I know about Terry, she works really hard and I'm sure you wouldn't allow someone to apply for promotion unless they had a competitive application. Based on Terry's application materials, I do not see how I can endorse her application." The dean explained there had been some staff turnover in her office with student interns picking up some of the slack over the past 3 months. She said she would personally overnight her copy of Terry's complete application for promotion to professor. The next day I received three, 3-inch binders that included clear evidence of Terry's publishing accomplishments and presented an independent trajectory of national and internationally recognized research, teaching innovations, and leadership on university and professional organizations. With such clear evidence that Terry met or exceeded the criteria for professor, I was able to write a very strong endorsement of Terry's application to the rank of professor. She received her promotion 6 months later and sent a nice thank-you note and a $5 gift card for coffee for supporting her successful application. I never mentioned to Terry the difficult document I almost had to write.

REFERENCES

de Lazari-Radek, K., & Singer, P. (2017). *Utilitarianism: A very short introduction*. Oxford, UK: Oxford University Press.

Fagermoen, M. S. (1997). Professional identity: Values embedded in meaningful nursing practice. *Journal of Advanced Nursing, 25*(3), 434–441. doi:10.1046/j.1365-2648.1997.1997025434.x

Peck, S. M. (2003). *The road less traveled, 25th anniversary edition: A new psychology of love, traditional values and spiritual growth*. New York, NY: Simon & Schuster.

Solomon, L. J., & Rothblum, E. D. (1984). Academic procrastination: Frequency and cognitive-behavioral correlates. *Journal of Counseling Psychology, 31*(4), 503–509. doi:10.1037/0022-0167.31.4.503

APPENDIX 9.1 ANNOTATED RECOMMENDATION LETTER FOR AN ACADEMIC POSITION

Natasha Fatale, PhD, RN
Professor and Chair of Facutly Search **Committee**
College of Nursing, Whatsamatta University

Write to a specific person – chair of the search committee, dean. Avoid writing to "Search Committee" or "To Whom It May Concern"

[Date]

Dear Dr. Fatale,

(Explain the purpose of the letter.)

I am writing as a professional reference in support of Dr. Rocket J. Squirrel's application for a faculty position at the College of Nursing at Whatsamatta University. I have known Dr. Squirrel for approximately 10 years as a supervisor, mentor, and collaborator. I first met Dr. Squirrel when he enrolled in the PhD program at Bob University and was appointed as a Graduate Research Assistant within the College of Nursing's Center for Nursing Research. As the Research Dean of the College at the time, I supervised Dr. Squirrel in his role and recognized his interest and ability to conduct research and pursue a scholarly academic career. During his tenure at the University, Dr. Squirrel was involved in a number of faculty research projects that resulted in **grant proposals, presentations, and publications. This involvement offered Dr. Squirrel a variety of research experiences that have prepared him for a future as an academic scholar.**

(Provide a match of the candidate's qualifications and the expectations of the job.)

Finally, I have first-hand knowledge of Dr. Squirrel's drive and ability to be a scientist as a result of co-authoring two data-based publications and a scholarly presentation with him.

(Discuss any collaborations.)

Following graduation from Bob University in 2005, Dr. Squirrel has been a productive scholar at the College of Nursing and Health Sciences at the University of Pottsylvania. During his tenure at the University of Pottsylvania as an Assistant Professor, he has maintained a **scholarly trajectory** that has included consistently publishing and presenting the results of his research, receiving extramural funding, and participating in and directing research teams. As evidence of his scholarly productivity, Dr. Squirrel has authored nine publications in scholarly journals and made 22 presentations at local, regional, and national nursing and other health-related scientific conferences. Also, since his initial appointment at the University of Pottsylvania, he has been a principal investigator or member of a number of research teams who have received in excess of $120,000 in extramural support for various research projects.

(Academic positions commonly require evidence of scholarly productivity. The criteria I have defined for scholarly productivity include consistently publishing and presenting the results of research, receiving extramural funding, and participating in and directing research teams.)

He is dedicated to developing a program of research through extramural support that focuses on developing innovative and culturally relevant interventions to improve access to care and appropriate utilization of healthcare resources.

(I provided an idea of his future areas of scholarly interest.)

Dr. Squirrel has made these significant scholarly contributions at the University of Pottsylvania while being an **effective teacher and fulfilling the service role of an Assistant Professor.** He has maintained a substantial teaching load that has included graduate and undergraduate courses, the content of which have been consistent with his research trajectory. He has regularly received above average to excellent student evaluations of his classroom teaching. The courses he has taught have included Global Perspectives in Health: Intersection of Equity, Economics and Culture, Health Disparities, and Social and Behavioral Determinants of Health. **This consistency between his research expertise and teaching allows Dr. Squirrel to deliver the most relevant evidence-based content to his students built upon his active program of research.** He has also contributed his scholarly expertise with access to care among underserved populations to various **service activities** within the university and the community. Of particular note is his appointment as a member of Pottsylvania Health Policy Forum Planning Committee and an advisor to the Uncle Dewlap Scholars program within the university.

Two other criteria I defined for an academic position include teaching and service.

Evidence that supports content expertise in teaching.

Service to the university and the community is another criterion of an academic position.

In addition to Dr. Squirrel's proven record of accomplishment as an emerging scholar and teacher and his involvement in service, he possesses several personal attributes that enrich his potential to be an outstanding faculty. I have observed him to be accountable to his coworkers and students, consistently completing tasks on or before deadlines. He can work independently with minimal direction, and anticipate and solve problems independently, only asking for direction when appropriate. Finally, and most importantly, Dr. Squirrel is a good "academic citizen" who happily takes on more than his share of teaching and service responsibilities for the greater good of the institution and the students. **Therefore, based on my professional collaborations and knowledge of Dr. Squirrel's research, teaching, and service productivity, I strongly recommend Dr. Squirrel's application for a faculty position in the College of Nursing, at Whatsamatta University.** If I can be of any further assistance please feel free to contact me.

Always provide a recommendation—good, bad, or lukewarm—for the position

Sincerely,

Bullwinkle J. Moose, PhD, RN
Bob University, College of Nursing
Frostbite Falls, Minnesota

APPENDIX 9.2 ANNOTATED RECOMMENDATION FOR TENURE AND PROMOTION

Betty Rubble, PhD, RN
Dean, College of Nursing
Bedrock University

Dear Dean Rubble,

Thank you for inviting me to review Dr. Fredrick Flintstone's application materials for promotion to the rank of Associate Professor with tenure within the College of Nursing at Bedrock University. **This document is to provide my evaluation of the originality and creativity of Dr. Flintstone's teaching and scholarship, as well as my assessment of the significance and impact of his work.**

> This is the exact language from the letter Dean Rubble sent me requesting I provide an evaluation of Dr Flintstone. Notice how the request identified only two areas for me to review and requests my assessment of the significance and impact. Thus, I need to establish the criteria for measuring significance and impact.

Since Dr. Flintstone was appointed Assistant Professor in the School of Nursing at Bedrock University in 2005, **I have been in contact with him through attending the same conferences and professional events. For 4 years prior to his appointment at Bedrock University, I was Dr. Flintstone's dissertation advisor when he was a doctoral student in the School of Nursing at Whatsamatta University. As a result of being Dr. Flintstone's advisor, I have co-authored two data-based publications in 2005 and 2006 and co-authored a scholarly presentation with him in 2006.**

> Discuss the duration and nature of my personal and professional relationship with the person I am evaluating and recommending.

Within Dr. Flintstone's application materials is a description of the innovations he has introduced to his teaching, quantitative and qualitative student evaluations of his classroom teaching, and three peer reviews of his classroom teaching. Dr. Flintstone's materials indicate he has taught five different courses during the past 5 years exclusively in the undergraduate nursing program. **There is no evidence that he has taught in any graduate courses or has participated in any graduate capstone or dissertation committees. Dr. Flintstone provides evidence that he has completely revised NUS402 "Community Health Nursing" including updating the reading assignments and rewriting the syllabus, all in-class lectures, and the final examination for the course. Of particular note is his innovation of developing a problem-based learning assignment that involves the students in this course collaborating with students from the School of Social Work to develop innovative health promotion programs for underserved communities in**

> If some critical component is not included I can only say it wasn't included in the materials I was provided.

> This section describes evidence of innovations in teaching.

the area. Dr. Flintstone also presents evidence that he has integrated his program of research into the course content of NURS332 "Health Care Technologies." As a requirement of this course, Dr. Flintstone assigns students to identify a novel use of the electronic health record (EHR), which he is installing and testing in the School of Nursing's Simulation Laboratory. Dr. Flintstone explains this assignment results in his students developing an understanding of the potential and the limitations of EHR technology as a platform for supporting healthcare delivery.

Dr. Flintstone's student and peer evaluations demonstrate a steady increase in classroom teaching competency. During his initial semester of teaching NURS201 and NURS402, his overall student quantitative teaching evaluations ranged from 2.8 to 3.5, below the school average of 3.8. Student qualitative evaluations from this semester included "He is an enthuastic teacher but seems disorganized . . . His lecture seems to be right out of the book." As a result of consultations with the Center on Educational Excellence and mentoring from senior faculty, Dr. Flintstone's student evaluations in the most recent academic year have ranged from 3.5 to 4.2, which is consistent with the faculty averages. As well, the student qualitative comments now reflect a more competent classroom presence, including "I like Dr. Flintstone's approach to teaching. He expects us to come to class prepared to discuss the readings and not just to take notes on his lecture . . . He knows his stuff. When asked a question he doesn't know, he looks up the answer on the break or by the next class."

> This section presents evidence indicating improvements in student quantitative and qualitative evaluations.

These current above-average student teaching evaluations are consistent with Dr. Flintstone's three most recent peer evaluations. In particular, Dr. Pearl Slaghoople attended Dr. Flintstone's lecture on personal health technologies in NURS332. Dr. Slaghoople commented that Dr. Flintstone exhibited outstanding 7/7 knowledge of the content, creativity, and management of the classroom. Dr. Slaghoople recomended Dr. Flintstone try different strategies to engaging all students in the discussion and be mindful that breaks every hour facilitate student learning. Dr. Slaghoople concluded by stating, "Overall Dr. Flintstone is an enthuastic, knowledgable instructor who effectively communicates with students and challenges them to use the knowledge aquired in their reading in new ways. He is a true asset to the faculty and students at BU."

> Evidence of peer evaluations indicating teaching competency.

Dr. Flintstone's scholarship over the past 5 years has involved installing and testing an EHR within the School of Nursing's Simulation Laboratory. This scholary work has resulted in interdiscplinary collaborations, extramural funding, peer-reviewed publications, and presentations at national and international meetings. Dr. Flintstone has collaborated with faculty from the School of Engineering as well as industry partner George N. Slate from Slate Health Technologies. Evidence from Dr. Flintstone's application materials indicates he has been the principal investigator or co-investigator on a number of extramural sources of support. Dr. Flinstone is the principal investigator on the current project titled "Reducing staff anxiety and resistance to learning a new EHR program." This project is funded by the National Science Foundation for 3 years for $256,000 and involves collaborations with an interdiscplinary team

> These are the criteria I set for originality and creativity in scholarship.

and personnel from Slate Health Technologies. During his tenure at Bedrock University, Dr. Flintstone has published as first author three data-based manuscripts in respected peer-reviewed journals including *Health Policy and Technology* and *Nursing Outlook*. In addition, Dr. Flintstone is a co-author on an additional five manuscripts in peer-reviewed journals. **Finally, over the previous 5 years, Dr. Flintstone has presented as first author the results of his scholarly activities at five scientific meetings, including the annual National Information Technology conference and the International Innovations in Medicine conference. He has also been a co-author on an additional eight presentations at regional, national, and international scientific conferences.**

Evidence of presentations at national and international conferences.

This evidence of originality and creativity indicates that Dr. Flintstone has had a significant impact on teaching and scholarship while at the College of Nursing at Bedrock University. Dr. Flintstone has created original and innovative teaching materials and scholarly deliverables. **Based on this evidence, I strongly endorse Dr. Flintstone's application for promotion to the rank of Associate Professor with tenure.**

Clear recommendation.

Thank you for the opportunity to review Dr. Flintstone's application materials and please let me know if I can be of any service in the future.

Greta Gazoo, PhD, RN
Professor of Nursing Health Technologies

APPENDIX 9.3 ANNOTATED RECOMMENDATION FOR MERIT BASED UPON ANNUAL REVIEW

Leonard Briscoe, PhD, RN
Assistant Professor, Psych Mental Health Nursing

Dr. Briscoe,

Explain the purpose of the letter.

The purpose of this letter is to provide a merit recommendation for 2017 based upon a review of your work product, performance, or productivity that you provided in your annual workload file. I am conducting this review in my

Explain the source of the information that was reviewed.

role as the Chair of the Faculty Annual Merit Committee according to the Faculty Bylaws listed in the Faculty Handbook. The contents of this file were compared with the criteria for the rank of Assistant Professor provided in the Faculty Handbook. This letter includes an evaluation

Explain why this document is being created and the relationship with the person being reviewed.

Explain the categories of work products, performance, and productivity that will be evaluated. This list will provide the ordering of the next paragraphs.

of **your teaching, research, and service activities** during 2017 and **based on comparing these activities with the criteria for rank, a merit recommendation is made.**

Explain how the recommendation will be made.

Provide a brief introduction to work history at the institution.

You were appointed to the rank of Assistant Professor in August 2015 and the following review is of your work products, performance, or productivity contained in your annual workload file during the 2017 calendar year. The criteria for teaching at the rank of Assistant Professor states "developing innovative approaches to knowledge dissemination within and outside the classroom along with improving student teaching evaluations that approach the mean of the faculty within the unit."

State the objective criteria by which work activities are being evaluated.

During Spring 2017 you taught three courses; a 1-day-per-week clinical course to 10 students (NUR237, Adult Acute Care Clinical), a three-credit-hour didactic course to 25 students (NUR344, Epidemiology) and a three-credit-hour online course to 23 students (NUR350, Ethics and Health Care Implications). During summer 2017 you taught the three-credit-hour NUR250 Addictive Behavior in Society to 18 students. Your student teaching evaluation scores for these courses **(overall mean = 3.81)** have improved over the scores you received in 2016 to a level consistent with the mean of the College of Nursing undergraduate faulty (mean = 3.7).

Evidence of student evaluations above the unit mean.

Your annual workload file indicates you have incorporated a discussion blog into your online course and the evaluations indicate this innovation is well received by your students.

Evidence of innovation.

As well, a number of student comments indicate that you are an enthusiastic instructor who is willing to answer students' questions, stimulates a lively interaction in your online course, and also returns assignments in a timely manner. Based on this evidence, your performance in teaching meets the standard of an Assistant Professor. **I recommend you continue to innovate and provide a high quality level of teaching in clinical, didactic, and online courses. Further, I recommend you include in your annual workload file student teaching evaluations from courses you taught during fall 2017.**

Provide recommendations for the future.

The criteria for research at the rank of Assistant Professor states "conducting an ongoing program of research, disseminating research findings in refereed publications, and national and international meetings." During 2017 you engaged in research activities by publishing as first author a manuscript titled "An intervention to positively change attitudes about vegetables among school-age children" in *the Journal of Pediatric Nursing*.

Objective criteria by which performance will be judged.

Evidence to support dissemination of findings in referred publications.

You have a second manuscript under review titled "Using social media to increase physical activity among middle school students" in the *Journal of Public Health Care Nursing*.

Evidence of an ongoing program of research.

Also, during 2017 you were conducting a study funded in 2016 for $5,000 by a University Research Scholarship to develop a healthy eating intervention using social media. You presented the preliminary findings of this study as a podium presentation at the State Nurses Convention in October 2017. Conducting preliminary research, publishing a manuscript, and presenting research at a state conference are consistent with meeting the standard of

Evidence of disseminating findings at a state-level meeting.

Provide an assessment as to if the performance aligns with the criteria.

(Provide recommendation for the future.) an Assistant Professor. I recommend you continue to publish your research, present your findings at national and international meetings, involve students in your research projects, and apply for larger extramural sources of funding to support your future research studies.

(Objective criteria by which performance will be judged.) The service criteria for the rank of Assistant Professor include "serving as committee member on PhD Dissertations, serving on college and university committees, and being involved in select professional organizations." Based on the materials in your annual workload file you were a member of the Skills Laboratory Redesign Task Force during 2017 that submitted recommendations for redesigning the skills laboratory for online learning. *(Evidence supporting serving on a college committee.)* Your annual workload file does not document your service on any PhD Dissertations or any service to the university or *(Provide an evidence-based recommendation.)* the profession during 2017. Based upon this evidence that you have not participated on PhD committees or university or professional service, your service activities appear to fall below the criteria for the standard for Assistant Professor. I recommend you participate in standing committees within *(Recommendation about how to work toward meeting the objective criteria.)* the school and the university and explore contributing service to professional organizations that would benefit from your expertise.

Based upon my evaluation of your teaching, research, and service activities documented in your annual workload file compared to the criteria for Assistant Professor during 2017, the merit recommendation of **"Meets the Standard" is applied.** Finally, if you have *(Provide a clear final recommendation that addresses the purpose of the letter.)* ambitions of being promoted to Associate Professor, your teaching, research, and service activities will need to be consistent with the criteria for this rank.

Meets the Standard for Assistant Professor
Jack McCoy, PhD, RN
Professor, Chair of the Faculty Annual Merit Committee

APPENDIX 9.4 ANNOTATED GRIEVANCE OR APPEAL LETTER

To: Adam Schiffe, JD, PhD, RN
Department Chair, Psych Mental Health Nursing

Cc: Jack McCoy, PhD, RN
Professor, Chair of the Faculty Annual Merit Committee

(If you are not writing the appeal to the person who provided the initial evaluation and recommendation Please keep them informed of what you are doing so they do not feel disenfranchised from the process.) Dear Dr. Schiffe,

The purpose of this letter to is to appeal the recommendation provided in my annual merit evaluation conducted by Jack McCoy, PhD. Dr. McCoy provided his evaluation and recommendation of my performance during the 2017 calendar year, which included his assessment of my work products, performance, or productivity. Dr. McCoy based his recommendation by comparing the materials included in my annual workload file kept in your office with the criteria for the rank of Assistant Professor provided in the Faculty Handbook. **The reason I am requesting this appeal** is because a number materials were not included or not fully interpreted in my file at the time of Dr. McCoy's review and that may have impacted his evaluation and recommendation.

State the reason you are requesting the appeal. Provide the reader with some new information or an alternative interpretation that would justify them reconsidering their initial evaluation and recommendation.

I agree with significant sections of Dr. McCoy's evaluation. He has accurately documented my teaching evaluations for spring and summer 2017, which have improved over my teaching evaluation scores for 2016. Dr. McCoy also mentioned my successful record of publishing a peer reviewed manuscript and presenting the preliminary results of my pilot work at the State Nurse's Convention during 2017. Finally, I will attempt to follow Dr. McCoy's recommendation for teaching, research, and service activities.

State points of agreement with the initial evaluation.

At the time of Dr. McCoy's evaluation, a number of materials were not available that may have impacted his initial evaluation and recommendation. As you know, I taught three courses in fall 2017 and, as the attachments indicate, my teaching evaluation scores for two of those three courses were well above the mean for faculty in our department. These teaching evaluations from all 2017 were not included in Dr. McCoy's evaluation. Dr. McCoy was also unaware that on December 10, 2017, I submitted, as principal investigator, a proposal to the Green & Cassidy Foundation to fund a project titled "Healthy communities form healthy foods" with a budget of $35,000. As well, Dr. McCoy perhaps misinterpreted that on December 13, 2017, I received notification that my manuscript titled "Using social media to increase physical activity among middle school students" was accepted and no longer under review for publication in the *Journal of Public Health Care Nursing*. **I have attempted to participate on the University Senate by being nominated to the faculty committee ballot although I was not elected. I have recently agreed to be a member of Olivia Benson's dissertation committee providing my expertise in social media. Finally, during the 2017 annual meeting of the Association of Pediatric Nurses, I volunteered to be on the media relations committee.**

Provide a detailed description about new information that was not initially considered in the evaluation.

Evidence of additional service at the university and to the profession.

Based upon materials that were not available or fully interpreted in Dr. McCoy's evaluation and recommendation, I am requesting that you reconsider the initial evaluation and recommendation of my annual merit evaluation for 2017. **These additional materials now included in my annual workload file appear consistent with a merit rating of "Exceeds the Standard" rather than "Meets the Standard."** Thank you for your kind consideration.

Formally ask the reviewer what you want as a result of your appear and provide rationale for why you are making this request.

Respectfully,
Leonard Briscoe, PhD, RN
Assistant Professor, Psych Mental Health Nursing

CHAPTER 10

REACHING READERS: OPEN ACCESS JOURNALS, INSTITUTIONAL REPOSITORIES, AND SOCIAL MEDIA

Amanda Y. Makula and Joseph Perazzo

PERSONAL STORY

As an academic librarian, I routinely witness the impact of making information available online on individual lives and on society. It is commonplace now to Google someone's name before meeting them in real life whether for a date, a job interview, or just out of curiosity. Your online identity is often readily available to anyone who decides to search for it, and it may help (or hinder) you in a variety of ways. In a positive example, I recall a time that an undergraduate student made his research project openly accessible online. He shared its link on his application to Harvard Medical School and watched excitedly as it received downloads from people at the institution. (Yes, he was accepted!) There are other instances when timing or circumstances make sharing information ill-advised or even dangerous. Another student who had written a critique of one of President Trump's campaign speeches disseminated the paper online, but when she graduated and was set to enter the military, she asked for help to take down her critique. She feared potential retaliation from fellow troops or commanders. In this situation, having her work publicly accessible was deemed risky. Stories like these help illustrate the complexity of sharing your work via a public venue. What might be appropriate in one situation could look very different in another.

INTRODUCTION

The purpose of this chapter is to introduce you to the landscape of open, online information sharing and educate you about some of the important considerations to take into account as you navigate your choices. I will introduce the open access movement, discuss its evolution, and explain what it can mean for you and your work. We will look at three main venues for sharing your work openly—open access journals, institutional repositories, and social media—and explore the benefits and complexities of each. Pay close attention to the critical decisions you will need to make depending on which platform you choose. Along the way, you will also develop an open access vocabulary and discover the importance of writing clearly and succinctly for a specific audience, be it academics, other nurses, patients, or the public.

THE LANDSCAPE OF OPEN, ONLINE INFORMATION SHARING

The previous chapters have discussed the publishing opportunities you might pursue as a student or a new faculty member. The traditional scholarly publishing system typically culminates in new knowledge being disseminated in the form of a journal article. Journals have been used to collect scientific works since a time when people did not use telephones, let alone Twitter. Journals were a way to have a meeting of the minds, open work up to argument and critique, and allow scientific advances to emerge.

Today, many journals are quite expensive, and their primary subscribers are not individuals but institutions. Academic libraries devote large portions of their budgets to journal subscriptions, purchasing some titles individually and others as part of packaged bundles. Through these subscriptions, libraries provide access to their own communities: faculty, staff, administration, and students. Thus, if you are enrolled at or employed by a college or university, you enjoy access to a wealth of information unavailable to those outside the academy, at least not without paying for it. Surely you can think of a time when you have Googled a topic and found an article you wanted to read only to discover that the only way to view it was to get out your credit card and pay for it.

Now, think for a moment about nurses. Upon graduation, many nurses are clinical practitioners without an institutional academic affiliation. Unless their employer pays for access to peer-reviewed research in the field, the nurses must pay for this access themselves or go without. Moreover, nurses are not acculturated to read scientific publications or participate in journal clubs; instead, they receive updates on the state of the science through continuing education, unit-based training, and/or certifications. The result is a world where even those who were once a part of the academy—and whose effective-ness in their jobs would certainly benefit from engagement with new developments in their various fields—are not regularly exposed to the majority of scholarly writing and research. But, times are changing, and the Internet has dismantled this barrier and increased the transparency of scientific discovery.

Enter *open access* (OA). In the late 20th century, the Internet and World Wide Web paved the way for the unrestricted electronic dissem-ination of information. This technology sparked revolutionary changes in research and knowledge distribution. (For a wonderful, entertaining introduction to open access, check out the short YouTube video "Open Access Explained!" by Nick Shockey and Jonathan Eisen at https://youtu.be/L5rVH1KGBCY.) One of the earliest examples of scientists sharing their research online is *arXiv.org*, a repository where physicists deposited prepublication versions (preprints, which is the version of an article prior to peer review) of their articles. The site has been incredibly active since its initial launch in 1991 and remains so to this day.

At the turn of the 21st century, the OA movement really took off. In 2000, the National Institutes of Health (NIH) launched PubMed Cen-tral, providing free access to the full text of some biomedical and life sciences literature. That same year, BioMed Central (BMC) published its first free article online. Today, BMC publishes over 300 open access, peer-reviewed journals (About BMC, n.d.). The Public Library of Science (PLoS) was founded a year later in 2001, "with a mission to accelerate progress in science and medicine by leading a transformation in research communication" (Who we are, n.d., para. 1). Then, in 2002, academics and leaders in the OA movement gathered in Budapest, Hungary, and penned the Budapest Open Access Initiative (Read the Budapest Open Access Initiative, n.d.), a global manifesto committing to open access to "accelerate research, enrich education, share the learning of the rich with the poor and the poor with the rich, make this literature as useful as it can be, and lay the foundation for uniting humanity in a com-mon intellectual conversation and quest for knowledge" (Chan et al., 2002, para. 1). For more significant dates in the evolution of open access, see Peter Suber's "Timeline of the Open Access Movement" at http://legacy.earlham.edu/~peters/fos/timeline.htm and the Open Access Directory's community wiki at http://oad.simmons.edu/oadwiki/Timeline.

Today, OA comes in a variety of forms, and authors may choose it for a variety of reasons. Some want as high a readership as possible, and there is evidence that open access articles enjoy a higher citation advantage than non-OA articles restricted by paywalls (Eysenbach, 2006; Norris, Oppenheim, & Rowland, 2008). Others are required by funding or institutional mandates to make their research openly available. (See the Registry of Open Access Repository Mandates and Policies [ROARMAP] at http://roarmap.eprints.org/ for an index of these mandates by type and country.) Some scholars want to ensure their work is accessible internationally, especially to scholars in developing and low-income countries who may not have institutional or personal access to expensive research literature. A commitment to OA is a commitment to fostering a more equitable system of information exchange. When viewed through a social justice lens, OA seeks to reduce disparities between those who are privileged with ready access to research and scholarship and those who are not (Alperin, Fischman, & Willinsky, 2008; Arunachalam, 2017; Musakali, 2010). Regardless of the underlying rationale for choosing OA, there are important considerations for just what *type* of open access is most appropriate in any particular situation. It is imperative to be mindful of the audience to whom you are writing; every publication venue—whether scholarly or popular—targets a specific group of readers. While it would be convenient to reach large and diverse populations by issuing your work in only one form, in reality, it does not work that way. Rather, disseminating your work using different methods and avenues, each appropriate to different audiences, is more effective than a singular approach.

OPEN ACCESS JOURNAL PUBLISHING

Some academic journals are fully open access; all the articles they publish are freely available to anyone. Other journals are "hybrids," giving authors the choice of whether or not they want their articles to be made openly available. Both types of OA journals may charge authors a fee (an *APC* or *article processing charge*), which can range from a few hundred dollars to a few *thousand*, in exchange for making the article openly accessible. The following list gives you a sense of some of the current open access journals in the field of nursing and their APCs:

- *Online Journal of Nursing Informatics* (http://www.himss.org/ojni) charges no APC

- *SAGE Open Nursing* (http://journals.sagepub.com/home/son) charges an APC of $445

- *AJN: American Journal of Nursing* (https://journals.lww.com/ajnonline/pages/default.aspx) charges an APC of $4,000

As you can see, it is important to familiarize yourself with a journal's options and policies for authors prior to submitting your work. It is equally important to ask yourself what *you* need from the deal. After all, your work is your intellectual property. As the Scholarly Publishing and Academic Resources Coalition (SPARC) explains, "as the author, you are the copyright holder unless and until you transfer the copyright to someone else in a signed agreement" (Author Rights, 2006). A "signed agreement" usually takes the form of a *copyright transfer agreement*, a contract that a publisher asks you to sign when your work is accepted for publication. Ask yourself: What rights, as the author, do you want to retain?

- Do you want the right to post your article on your own website?
- Share copies with classmates or colleagues?
- Present your findings at a conference?

Does the publisher allow you to do those things, or does the publisher claim exclusive copyright to your work and its reproduction, distribution, and modifications? Before submitting your article, look for this information on the journal's website. It is often located in the information for authors section or the submission guidelines. If you cannot find it, ask the publisher for it. Otherwise, you will see it spelled out when your article is accepted and you are presented with the copyright transfer agreement. Read the fine print on this agreement closely. By signing the agreement, what rights are you granting the publisher? What rights, if any, do you retain? If you do not agree to the contract's terms, you can try to re-negotiate them with the publisher. For example, SPARC developed an Author Addendum—a "legal instrument that modifies the publisher's agreement and allows you to keep key rights to your articles"—specifically for this purpose (Author Rights, 2006). Fill it out, attach it to the contract, and present it to the publisher.

An advantage of choosing to publish with an OA journal is that the terms of the publishing agreement are generally author-friendly, allowing you to retain key rights without petitioning for them in special negotiations as described previously.

Now you may be wondering how to find OA journals in your field that are a good match for your work. You can start by consulting resources that curate information about journals, such as Ulrichsweb Global Serials Directory. Many academic libraries purchase this online subscription database. It allows you to search for journals fitting specific criteria, including subject area, language, and yes, OA options. Ulrichsweb gives you details like who publishes the journal and in what country, a description of its content, and a link to the publisher's website. Look for Ulrichsweb in your library's online database listing. The Directory of Open Access Journals (DOAJ), "a community-curated online directory that indexes and provides access to high quality, open access, peer-reviewed journals," is another source to explore (https://doaj.org). This directory allows you to filter journals by subject area, APC requirement, peer review presence, and so forth. Finally, do not hesitate to ask a librarian for assistance. Many universities have a librarian who specializes in scholarly communication and can help you navigate questions about open access publishing.

A word of caution: As you survey the OA publishing landscape, you need to know that not all OA journals are legitimate. Some OA journals are referred to as *predatory publishers*. These are unethical publishers that seek to profit from APCs without providing the publishing services they promise to deliver. In their article, "Selecting an Open Access Journal for Publication: Be Cautious," Hoffecker, Hastings-Tolsma, Vincent, and Zuniga (2016) provide an excellent overview for nursing students and clinicians of the benefits—and potential pitfalls—of publishing with an OA journal. Determining whether a journal is disreputable is complex and requires critical thinking, but some common "red flags" include:

- Aggressive article solicitation (often by email spam)
- Very fast article acceptance (a sign that the lengthy process of peer review has not been employed)
- Disclosure of an APC only after article acceptance
- Fake information (e.g., names of editorial board members who do not actually serve or even exist)

Fortunately, there are resources that can help you discern the bona fide from the bogus. Together with the DOAJ, the Committee on Publication Ethics (COPE; https://publicationethics.org/), the Open Access Scholarly Publishers Association (OASPA; https://oaspa .org/), and the World Association of Medical Editors (WAME; http:// www.wame.org/) have come together to create "Principles of Transparency and Best Practice in Scholarly Publishing" (Redhead, 2018). The publishers and editors listed on these organizations' membership rosters have passed rigorous quality control standards and have agreed to an ethical code of conduct. Another excellent guide is "Think Check Submit" (https://thinkchecksubmit.org/), a tutorial created by COPE, DOAJ, OASPA, and other respected organizations. This resource walks you through the process of evaluating a journal's suitability for publishing your work.

Ultimately, even if you do not publish your work in an OA journal or you decide not to seek formal publication at all, you may still want to share it widely. Fortunately, you have other options for distributing the new knowledge you have developed.

OPEN ACCESS INSTITUTIONAL REPOSITORIES

In all likelihood, your college or university has an institutional repository (IR). It may also be referred to as an open access repository, digital repository, online archive, or digital archive. The IR stores, preserves, and provides free access to content produced at the institution including faculty and student scholarship. Prior to the adoption of IRs, much of this content never reached an audience beyond the walls of the institution. However, today, if you want to ensure that your work is permanently preserved and made available worldwide to students, faculty, researchers, clinicians, and the general public—anyone with an Internet connection, in fact—then the IR is an excellent vehicle to achieve that.

Posting your scholarship in the IR provides several benefits. First, it means your work will be affiliated with your university, which lends it greater credibility (good for you) and raises the profile of your school (good for the institution). The IR also helps your work find an audience. For example, the IR at my institution, which currently uses the Digital Commons platform administered by bepress, cooperates with search engines such as Google so that its content is "crawled" and indexed, and thus discoverable, to people conducting searches on the Internet. In other words, no one has to know about the IR to discover your work. Instead, they can find it just by typing keywords into an Internet search engine! And once someone finds your work, the IR supplies valuable readership information to you as an author. Depending on the specific IR platform that your university uses, you may have access to metrics, such as the number of times your work is downloaded, geolocation of where in the world those downloads originate, and even the organizational profile (commercial, educational, governmental, military, etc.), and specific URL domains of your readers.

Sounds good, right? By now you might be thinking "sign me up!" If you are interested in using the IR, there may already be an opportunity waiting for you at your academic institution. Typically, universities with an IR capture the electronic theses and dissertations (ETDs) produced by their graduate students. When you complete a master's or doctoral program, you can expect to receive instructions on how to participate in this process, which varies by institution. Some universities require students to upload their thesis or dissertation to *PQTD Global*, a subscription database produced by the commercial publisher ProQuest. This submission process may include an option for students to grant permission for a copy of the work to be added to the IR. Other universities require students to submit their thesis or dissertation directly to the IR and allow students to choose whether to send a copy to ProQuest. One of the main differences between the IR and ProQuest is that the former provides open access to your work so that anyone worldwide can find, read, and share it, whereas ProQuest provides access only to people who are affiliated with a subscribing institution, unless you as the author pay a fee to make your work open access (ProQuest Dissertation FAQ, n.d.). On the other hand, ProQuest provides a centralized database used by academics for searching and discovering ETDs on a particular topic. If you are curious about the policy at your institution, talk to your advisor or visit the graduate records office.

Regardless of whether you submit your thesis and/or dissertation to the IR or to ProQuest, you will be prompted with choices for either venue. These choices depend on your institution's policies and how it has decided to handle the preservation and dissemination of graduate student work. One option you may have is whether to *embargo* your work. Placing an embargo on your work restricts access to its full text for the period of time you specify. For example, if you apply an embargo of one year, then the full text of your thesis or dissertation will not be available to viewers until one year from the date it is posted. Typically, the metadata (title, abstract, and other information about the work) is unaffected by an embargo and therefore remains openly available.

You may be wondering why you would want to apply an embargo. After all, you want as many people to read your work as possible! Indeed, many students do not choose an embargo. However, there are circumstances where it might make good sense to employ an embargo on your scholarly work. For example, if you are also submitting your work, or a close derivative of it, for publication elsewhere, it is a good idea to find out what the publisher's policies are regarding previous publication and whether they classify inclusion in an IR as a previous publication of the work. Another situation where an embargo might be appropriate is if your research contains a pending patent or private information about subjects such as medical data although in that case, redaction or not including the information is likely more appropriate than an embargo. If you are not sure whether to restrict access to your work by applying an embargo, start a conversation about it with your advisor or reference librarian.

In addition to an embargo option, you may have a choice to attach a *Creative Commons (CC) license* to your work. A CC license lets you specify to others how they may re-use your work going forward. The most basic and accommodating license is CC BY, which allows others to "distribute, remix, tweak, and build upon your work, even commercially, as long as they credit you for the original creation" (About the licenses, n.d.). Alternatively, perhaps you want to stipulate that your work may only be used noncommercially, without monetary gain. In that case, you may wish to apply the CC BY-NC (Attribution-Noncommercial) license. There are six licenses available (Figure 10.1), and you may have the opportunity to apply one at the point you submit your work. In the IR at my institution, for example, there is a field with a drop-down menu that lists the six licenses, and students or faculty simply select which one (if any) they want to attach to their work. Then, when the thesis or dissertation is posted, the license and its machine readable technology will display on the record for human users, search engines, and software systems alike.

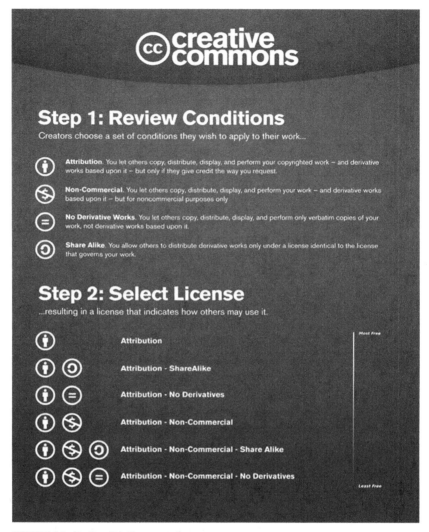

FIGURE 10.1 Six Creative Commons licenses.

Source: Image obtained at https://wiki.creativecommons.org/images/a/a4/Creativecommons-how-to-license
-poster_eng.pdf and used in accordance with the Creative Commons Attribution 4.0 International license.

SOCIAL MEDIA

So far, you have been learning about sharing your scholarly writing via
scholarly platforms, such as peer-reviewed journals and institutional
repositories. These avenues are invaluable for clinical nurses or nurses
pursuing academic degrees. However, the landscape of scholarly dissemination is changing. Gone are the days when one had to "hit the
stacks," using print indexes to find an obscure article buried somewhere
in the darkest corners of the library. The Internet, along with countless
apps and programs available on smartphones, notebooks, and tablets,
has made it possible for people to obtain and explore information in a

matter of seconds. Likewise, academics now have access to social media that can disseminate their work to vastly larger audiences than they are able to reach with traditional (non-OA) journals, and they are capitalizing on the Internet's power to get their work out to a wider audience. In this section, I discuss the nature of social media and how you might leverage these as a form of scientific dissemination.

Social media include a multitude of web-based programs that allow people to connect, communicate, and collaborate with each other online. You may have noticed that more and more professional organizations are aligning themselves with social media to increase their ability to follow trends, find target populations, and communicate with the public. One of the challenges of using social media is keeping up with the ever-changing options and their platforms. As for-profit entities, social media companies constantly monitor the market and look for new ways to entice new users and expand their influence. New tools debut and existing ones disappear. Terms of service change. This impermanence is an important distinction between social media sites and institutional repositories, the latter of which is designed to preserve materials permanently. Social media is constantly evolving, and it is entirely possible that between the time of this writing and the point when this book is published, some platforms will be defunct or will have changed from their current iteration. Meanwhile, new social media tools will take their place. Miah (2017) inventories some of the top social media and niche tech tools used by academics. You are probably already familiar with LinkedIn, Skype, Twitter, WordPress, and YouTube. Less familiar social media include Authorea, hypothes.is, Kudos, Slack, or Zotero. These and many other tools can enhance your online professional presence and help your work be more widely accessed.

If you want to use social media, a great place to begin is to create a professional profile dedicated to discussing your work. Then, use the search features built into the sites to find and connect with people, organizations, advocacy groups, and events related to your work. In your profile, provide your "followers" with summaries of your work. Professional networking sites such as LinkedIn allow you to describe your writing and research projects. If you have published an article in an OA journal or have deposited it in an IR, include it in your profile and send out a link to it with an announcement like, "My work is featured in [JOURNAL] where I found that [OVERALL FINDINGS]" so that people can peruse it for themselves. If your contract with the publisher allows you to attach the full text, do that as well.

Always remember that by its very nature, social media is designed to disseminate short bursts of information quickly to a large audience. Keep your posts pithy and to the point. Attach a visual representation of your findings—an image, chart, or graph—if you have one. Capture attention with a provocative title or heading. Send out bullet points, summary statements, or surprising facts from your research. When you attend conferences, post pictures of your posters, "tweet" summary points from presentations, and reflect on what you have learned. (If something controversial happened and has people talking, share your take on it!) Above all, use plain language. You want people without a nursing background (patients, the public, family, and friends) to be able to understand and use the results of your work.

Although social media platforms offer a more flexible, informal avenue to communicate with readers than do traditional scholarly publications, you still need to play by the rules whenever you create a post. Do not plagiarize others' work. If you are using information or ideas from another source, put it into your own words and be sure to cite it. If something does not originate with you, lead your audience to the source by giving credit to the authors.

It takes some time to get off the runway, but social media can help you get the word out on your work and can help you make connections with others who share your interests. Next, we take a closer look at two popular social media tools for sharing academic scholarship: blogs and academic social networking sites.

BLOGS

Blogs are websites that are updated on a regular basis, and typically keep a continuous archive of posts that can be revisited. Blogs came onto the scene when people started building their own personal websites and were akin to personal diaries. People could post just about anything they wanted to post, and others could visit and follow the blog over time. Whether a person wants to share their day-to-day experiences, write about a favorite band or entertainer, chronicle their travels, or even document a journey through chemotherapy, blogs give people full liberty to write about what they want. Recently, corporations, popular publications, news outlets, and individual scientists have used blogs to share their current work and cutting-edge developments. By tagging their posts with keywords describing the content, bloggers find and connect with readers.

One of the key advantages to blogging is the freedom it provides. Blogging gives authors a tremendous amount of editorial freedom that they may not exercise in journals. For example, blogs take on a much more conversational tone than scientific articles. Authors can highlight aspects of their work in plain language and stimulate dialogue with an audience beyond academia. This latitude brings up a universally important point when it comes to the language you choose to use in any writing project. People who work in healthcare learn to speak a different language than the public, and nowhere is this more evident than in scholarly writing. Friends and family members may read your work and ask you to translate it into a language they can understand. While writing scholarly papers, authors often conform to terminology and sentence structure that is accepted or traditional among their peers or in their field of interest. Blogs, on the other hand, allow for the use of plain language. Authors can cast off their obligation to write a certain way and simply express their ideas as they see fit. This is nothing new to nurses, trained from day one to simplify complex topics to educate their patients. When patients in the hospital require education, nurses do not hand them the latest issue of a scientific journal and wish them happy reading. Why not? It is the *best* evidence, right? Perhaps, but it would be ridiculously ineffective because the writing was not designed to be read for the purpose of patient education.

Even when it comes to scholarly writing, you must always re-member that very real human beings are the ones reading your work. Whether an individual is a layperson or the top scientist in their field, most people are not only attracted to simple writing but also turned off by writing that is too complicated. Daniel Oppenheimer (2005) pub-lished research in *Applied Cognitive Psychology* titled, "Consequences of Erudite Vernacular Utilized Irrespective of Necessity: Problems With Using Long Words Needlessly." Spoiler alert: Using complicated language does not make you sound smart and, in fact, may have the opposite effect.

Another obligation that you can abandon while blogging is the effort to appear dispassionate or unbiased. Scholars are often trained to avoid implicit and explicit biases in their writing as bias can diminish the impact of the dissemination and possibly even appear prejudicial. When Joe began his postdoctoral fellowship, his mentor constantly pointed out his use of the word "unfortunately." At first, he did not understand what the big deal was. He would write something like, "Unfortunately, two participants did not seek out HIV care following their HIV test and advanced to AIDS prior to care initiation." Isn't that true? Isn't that unfortunate? Certainly, a person becoming ill is unfortunate, right? However, the point of the paper was to report on HIV care initiation, not to give his evaluation of or opinions on individual cases. With blogs, authors can express themselves more freely while still presenting valu-able evidence. Blogging allows you to combine research, clinical wisdom, personal evaluation, and reflection, all merged into one piece of writing.

The following story is a real-world example of how a blog can com-plement scientific scholarship. Joe published a study in a peer-reviewed journal. There were findings that did not fit into the mold of scientific articles, but he still had more to say about what he learned in the study. He was impressed by people with HIV who stepped in and offered help and guidance when they learned someone else had been diag-nosed. Joe heard these stories and wanted to share them. He contacted an online HIV patient resource portal that invited him to contribute a blog to their site. He wrote the post in Exhibit 10.1 to share this informa-tion with key stakeholders and to convey aspects of his work that did not make it into scientific articles.

EXHIBIT 10.1: PEOPLE WITH HIV: POSITIVELY POWERFUL

Reflecting on the discovery of HIV, we see a story of unprece-dented progress in medicine and society. While challenges remain and diligent scientific and social efforts continue, the story of HIV is one of fear, perseverance, hope, compassion, and courage. The progress we have seen is often credited almost exclusively to the innovative scientists and healthcare workers responsible for the research and development of treatments and even a cure for HIV. The societal contributions of their work cannot be understated— the renewed lives, the decrease in societal risk, and the possibility for people once thought hopeless to live long and healthy lives is largely due to their efforts.

However, we must never forget something very important: from the early days of the HIV epidemic, people with HIV have played a pivotal role in efforts to learn about the disease, discover new treat-ments, and provide love and social support to people diagnosed with HIV and their families. One can only imagine the fear of the un-known that accompanied participation in early clinical trials testing medications for HIV and the hope against hope that the drugs would work. While many did not live for us to hear their stories, we must always remember their contribution to the discovery of a solution to HIV infection. Furthermore, the courage of people with HIV to stand against ignorance and advocate for each other and for society continues to be a foundation that makes continued progress possible.

In my work, I have seen the impact that people living with HIV have on the successful linkage of newly diagnosed individuals to care. I completed a study in which I interviewed 30 people recently diagnosed with HIV about their experiences with learning about their HIV diagnosis and how they came to the decision to seek out help. While not everyone in the study had a friend or acquaintance with HIV, many of them did. They shared about the love, encour-agement, and hope they were given by people living with HIV. Whether in-person, on a long drive, on discussion boards, or in on-line chats, people with HIV shared their strength and experiences with these newly diagnosed men and women. Over and over, the participants told me, "they helped me realize that I needed to take action and start treatment." Their stories showed me just how cru-cial people with HIV are in the big picture; they do not just pro-vide relatable experiences, they help people get into care, even if by being a walking example of hope and survival. Today, I often

(continued)

> **EXHIBIT 10.1: PEOPLE WITH HIV: POSITIVELY POWERFUL (*continued*)**
>
> hear participants say, "I like participating in studies," rather than, "I hope it helps someone." If you are a person living with HIV, whether you participate in studies, volunteer, share your story, or simply live your life everyday as a living breathing miracle, you are helping the world more than you know; you are crucial; you are powerful. Thank you.

ACADEMIC SOCIAL NETWORKING SITES

You may have heard your classmates or professors mention Academia.edu or ResearchGate, two prominent *academic social networking sites* (ASNSs). These sites are a specialized form of social media targeting the higher education community. They encourage students, faculty, researchers, and scholars to upload their articles, network with others in the field, and peruse job opportunities. They provide usage analytics, such as how often your profile has been viewed or the number of times others have recommended your paper. (Depending on the specific service, access to certain features may require a paid subscription to the site.) Some academics enthusiastically use ASNSs, while others warn against them (Bond, 2017). There are a number of considerations to keep in mind as you explore ASNSs.

First, it is important to understand that ASNSs are for-profit sites. (Yes, the name Academia.edu is especially misleading.) They are not designed or hosted by educational or non-profit entities but instead were founded by venture capitalists and operated by for-profit companies. Even though their user base is faculty and researchers, they are more akin to Facebook than they are to institutional repositories. When you use them, you assume the same risks as with other online consumer activities: the potential for your information to be shared with third parties, to encounter ads or pop-ups, or to lose your paper and its usage statistics if the site eventually folds. I know it is not fun to wade through the legalese of a site's terms of service but if you want to know exactly what rights the site claims and what rights remain with you, it is a good idea to look.

ASNSs are attractive because they provide an easy avenue for making one's scholarship openly accessible online. If you do not have the time or tech skills to create your own website on which to host your articles, you can sign up for an account with an ASNS and immediately begin uploading your work. However, just because it is easy does not mean it is legal. Remember the copyright transfer agreements discussed earlier? In many cases, once you have signed a contract with a publisher, you no longer own the rights to your own work. This means that you legally cannot reproduce and distribute it via an ASNS or otherwise. Some users of Academia.edu found this out the hard way in 2013 when the publisher Elsevier issued takedown notices to the site for hosting articles violating the publisher's copyright (Howard, 2013). It happened again in 2017, though this time with ResearchGate, and on a much larger scale. Rather than targeting 3,000 articles for takedown, publishers, including Elsevier and the American Chemical Society, identified roughly *7 million* articles and filed a lawsuit against the site (Van Noorden, 2017). If you decide to use ASNSs, be sure to comply with the publisher's copyright policies. If you do not know the copyright policies of the journals with which you published your scholarship, check out SHERPA ROMEO (http://www.sherpa.ac.uk/romeo/search.php), an online site that tracks journal policies and author's rights as they relate to self-archiving. In many cases, you may be able to share the postprint / author's accepted manuscript (the version of the article after undergoing peer review but without the publisher's typesetting and formatting) even if the final publisher's PDF is not allowed.

If you *are* able to upload your articles, you can solicit feedback from readers on the site. You can also see how much traffic your work is getting by viewing its metrics, such as number of views. Of course, there are other ways besides uploading your articles that you can use ASNSs. If there is someone whose work interests you or aligns closely with your own, you can "follow" them to keep abreast of his or her latest work. Maybe you want to communicate with another author by sending a direct message, or to look for potential co-authors for a new project. In this way, ASNSs act as a virtual community for academia. While a professor may be the only expert in a field at his or her institution, using an ASNS connects the professor to other leading authorities across the world, facilitating the kind of networking that in the past could only happen infrequently at conferences and other professional gatherings.

For all the benefits that social media offers, the question becomes why more scholars do not take advantage of these tools. It is important to point out that while scholars are no longer strictly bound to scientific publications, these resources remain incredibly important. Peer review is a cornerstone of rigorous science. If someone sent me a scientific paper about the latest developments related to aerospace engineering, I would not be able to tell you if the paper was methodologically rigorous or accurate or if it was a pile of rubbish. It may be very interesting, and it may even sound plausible. I would smile, nod, and be stupefied by the foreign terms and concepts. That is why this area of scholarly writing needs to be reviewed by an aerospace engineer; that is, someone who can understand it. More importantly, it needs to be reviewed by someone within the field who can *evaluate* the merit of the content and validity of the science. Scholars want their work to make it into peer-reviewed journals (whether OA or not) alongside others in their field so they can make their contribution to knowledge in their area.

There are also the pragmatic considerations regarding the need to publish as part of many academic careers. As you have learned in this book, publishing is a compulsory component of job security for many people working in the university setting. While the expectations for publication varies across institutions and individual positions, regular dissemination of scholarly work is often necessary to be considered for re-appointment and tenure. In other words, scholars focus their efforts on scholarly writing because their jobs literally depend on it. Alas, I have never heard of anyone getting tenure based on his or her active presence on Twitter, nor have I heard of new care guidelines developed from a series of Facebook posts, blogs, or YouTube videos. You should never lose sight of the importance of scholarly writing for scientific journals. That said, I would encourage you not to underestimate the power of these online resources.

Another reason more scholars may not encourage students to use Facebook, Twitter, YouTube, or Blogger to disseminate their work is that they may not use these resources themselves. Despite some appearances to the contrary, not everyone uses social media daily. A number of people prefer to call or meet in person with friends to describe sushi they ate last night, rather than posting a picture of it on Facebook and checking to see how many "likes" they receive. People may not use social media for a host of reasons: They do not know how it works, do not feel they have time, they have misconceptions about it, or they just do not want to. Understandably, many are concerned about privacy issues. You may have heard about the Cambridge Analytica scandal wherein the company breached and exploited Facebook user data to create psychological profiles of users, target them with ad campaigns, and ultimately influence political elections (Cadwalladr & Graham-Harrison, 2018; Rosenberg, Confessore, & Cadwalladr, 2018). There is no denying, however, that we are in the Internet age. A click of a button taking less than a second can send a piece of information to thousands, even millions, of people. If you want to reach a vast audience quickly and easily, social media can be the right tool for the job.

CONCLUSION

This chapter introduced you to some of the key considerations in making your work openly available to an online audience. You learned about the history and rationale behind the OA movement. You contemplated an appropriate venue for sharing your work—open access journal, institutional repository, and/or social media—and some of the important choices and consequences that come with each, all within the context of nursing education and the profession. You now recognize terms like *APC*, *embargo*, *Creative Commons*, *copyright transfer agreement*, *predatory publishers*, and *academic social networking sites*, and understand their place within the OA landscape. With this new knowledge, you are ready to decide if and how you want to share your work with as wide an audience as possible in an instantaneous online environment. Good luck and have fun!

REFERENCES

About BMC. (n.d.) Retrieved from https://www.biomedcentral.com/about

About the licenses. (n.d.) Retrieved from https://creativecommons.org/licenses/

Alperin, J. P., Fischman, G., & Willinsky, J. (2008). Open access and scholarly publishing in Latin America: Ten flavours and a few reflections. *Liimc en Revista, 4*(2), 172–185. Retrieved from http://revista.ibict.br/liinc/article/view/3165/2831

Arunachalam, S. (2017). Social justice in scholarly publishing: Open access is the only way. *American Journal of Bioethics, 17*(10), 15–17. doi: 10.1080/15265161.2017.1366194

Author Rights. (2006). Using the SPARC author addendum. Retrieved from https://sparcopen.org/our-work/author-rights/brochure-html

Bond, S. (2017, January 23). Dear scholars, delete your account at Academia.edu. *Forbes.* Retrieved from https://www.forbes.com

Cadwalladr, C. & Graham-Harrison, E. (2018, March 17). Revealed: 50 million Facebook profiles harvested for Cambridge Analytica in major data breach. *The Guardian.* Retrieved from https://www.theguardian.com

Eysenbach, G. (2006). Citation advantage of open access articles. *PLoS Biology, 4*(5), 692–698. doi:10.1371/journal.pbio.0040157

Hoffecker, L., Hastings-Tolsma, M., Vincent, D., & Zuniga, H. (2016). Selecting an open access journal for publication: Be cautious. *The Online Journal of Issues in Nursing, 21*(1), 8. doi:10.3912/OJIN.Vol21No01PPT03

Howard, J. (2013, December 6). Posting your latest article? You might have to take it down. *Chronicle of Higher Education.* Retrieved from https://www.chronicle.com

Miah, A. (2017, March 9). The A to Z of social media for academia. *Times Higher Education.* Retrieved from https://www.timeshighereducation.com

Musakali, J. J. (2010, June 1). Bridging the digital divide through open access. *SciDevNet.* Retrieved from https://www.scidev.net/global/digital-divide/opinion/bridging-the-digital-divide-through-open-access.html

Norris, M., Oppenheim, C., & Rowland, F. (2008). The citation advantage of open-access articles. *Journal of the American Society for Information Science and Technology, 59*(12), 1963–1972. doi:10.1002/asi.20898

Oppenheimer, D. M. (2005). Consequences of erudite vernacular utilized irrespective of necessity: Problems with using long words needlessly. *Applied Cognitive Psychology, 20*(2), 139–156. doi:10.1002/acp.1178

ProQuest dissertation FAQ. (n.d.) Retrieved from http://www.proquest.com/products-services/dissertations/proquest-dissertations-faq.html#discovery

Read the Budapest open access initiative. (n.d.). Retrieved from http://www.budapestopenaccessinitiative.org/read

Redhead, C. (2018, January 15). Principles of transparency and best practice in scholarly publishing. Retrieved from https://oaspa.org/principles-of-transparency-and-best-practice-in-scholarly-publishing-3

Rosenberg, M., Confessore, N., & Cadwalladr, C. (2018, March 17). How Trump consultants exploited the Facebook data of millions. *New York Times.* Retrieved from https://www.nytimes.com

Van Noorden, R. (2017, October 10). Publishers threaten to remove millions of papers from ResearchGate. *Nature.* Retrieved from https://www.nature.com/news/publishers-threaten-to-remove-millions-of-papers-from-researchgate-1.22793

Who we are. (n.d.). Retrieved from https://www.plos.org/who-we-are

CHAPTER 11

GRAMMAR, SCIENTIFIC, DISSERTATION, CREDIBILITY

Carol J. Scimone

Dear Grammar Cop,

You are a (noun) and I hope you (verb) soon. Have a/an (adjective) day.

PERSONAL STORY

I have a confession to make; my name is Carol and I am a grammar cop. At least, I am a reformed grammar cop. When I was in college, I worked for a major international airline. One day, our station manager sent all employees a memo that contained a letter he had written to the Board of Airport Commissioners. There were numerous spelling and grammar errors, which were understandable because English was his second language. Trying to be proactive, or perhaps because I had just been accepted to the journalism program at the University of Southern California, I corrected all the errors and returned the memo to him. He was not amused. He sent the memo back to me with a giant "X" written in a thick, black marker, and covering the entire page. That was the day I entered grammar cop rehab.

INTRODUCTION

"I had someone correct my grammar once on a blind date, and within the first 10 minutes the date was over. You just do not correct somebody's grammar. That's just not okay. I'm from Tennessee, so I probably say everything wrong. I might have said 'ain't,' or something like that."

—Reese Witherspoon

The quote by Reece Witherspoon is only 49 words but speaks volumes about a controversy that has developed in the United States surrounding grammar. It is the virtual fisticuffs between one who uses poor grammar and another who feels it necessary to point out the errors. If you read the comment section of online articles from your local newspaper you will see it; a conversation that often goes something like this:

PERSON 1: There too stupid to know the difference.

PERSON 2: Before you condemn someone, perhaps look in the mirror. "There" should be "They're" (for *they are*) and "diference" is spelled "difference."

PERSON 1: Don't you have anything better to do than call me out for a few spelling mistakes, Homeskillet? Get a life!

PERSON 2: I would tell you to get a job, but with that vocabulary you are clearly not qualified to do anything other than asking me if I want fries with my burger.

Both may have a point. But this type of interaction is often highly charged and causes anger, hurt feelings, and ruffled feathers. Perhaps it is the public humiliation or the tone in which the so-called "grammar cop" delivers opinions, but such interactions are often not viewed as helpful. The grammar-challenged person is assumed to be ignorant while the grammar cop is seen simply as a snob.

This chapter provides you with unsolicited but commonly offered grammar advice. The first section discusses why grammar is important, particularly in scholarly writing. The next section discusses common errors that I have seen during my 6 years of editing dissertations and provides suggestions on how to remedy those errors. If you would like to know more about grammar, you will find a list of suggested reading at the end of this chapter. If you do not wish to know where the apostrophe is placed in a plural possessive, please find a good editor.

Why? Because you never know when you will run into a grammar cop. Perhaps it is the human resources manager to whom you sent your curriculum vitae. Or what about the editor of that journal in which you so desperately want your article to be published? Did you know that editor was an English major? Making mistakes in grammar, spelling, and punctuation can sometimes mean your hard work ends up in a shredder instead of in a journal.

THE REAL-WORLD GRAMMAR TEST

The founder and CEO of iFixit and Dozuki, Kyle Wiens, requires that every job applicant take a grammar test.

"Extenuating circumstances aside (dyslexia, English language learners, etc.), if job hopefuls cannot distinguish between "to" and "too," their applications go into the bin," Wiens writes (Wiens, 2012).

Wiens points out that iFixit is the world's largest online repair manual and Dozuki assists companies in writing their own technical documents, so grammar is an important part of many positions. He requires everyone to take the test, even those whose jobs do not include writing (Wiens, 2012).

Wiens is not alone. Early in my journalism career, I worked for a news director who would throw out the audition tapes of applicants who made any grammar or spelling errors in their cover letters and resumes, especially if they misspelled the news director's name. Like Wiens, my news director believed people who make few or no mistakes in grammar are likely to make fewer mistakes in their work. And like Wiens, my news director believed good grammar is relevant for all companies because *good grammar is credibility*.

When I use the term "grammar" in this writing, it means grammar, punctuation, and spelling. Punctuation is just as important as good grammar and a properly spelled word. For example, read the two sentences below.

> Original: I like cooking my family and my pets.

> Edited: I like cooking, my family, and my pets.

I am sure the author's family is happy he knows how to use commas and wasn't trying to put a modern twist on Hansel and Gretel.

When it comes to being fussy about grammar, people in certain professions need to have a more solid grasp of the English language than others. Reporters are just one example. Attorneys, professors, researchers, bloggers, in fact, anyone whose work involves writing or speaking should know not to splice commas, cause run-on sentences, or dangle their participles. They should also own a dictionary.

LANGUAGE FLUIDITY AND HOW THE PUBLIC INFLUENCES THE DICTIONARY

The English language is fluid, constantly changing to meet the needs of the times. Over the past several years, there has been an uproar over Merriam-Webster's definition of the word *literally*. Merriam-Webster.com defines *literally* as follows:

1: in a literal sense or manner: such as

    a: in a way that uses the ordinary or primary meaning of a term or expression • He took the remark *literally.* • a word that can be used both literally and figuratively b: used to emphasize the truth and accuracy of a statement or description • The party was attended by *literally* hundreds of people

c: with exact equivalence: with the meaning of each individual word given exactly • The term "Mardi Gras" *literally* means "Fat Tuesday" in French

d: in a completely accurate way • a story that is basically true even if not *literally* true

2 : in effect: virtually—used in an exaggerated way to emphasize a statement or description that is not *literally* true or possible • This will *literally* turn the world upside down.

So, it turns out, literally means both *literally* and *figuratively*.

A 2013 article on Salon.com argues that pop culture has a hand in the misuse of such words (Coleman, 2013). Rob Lowe's character on *Parks and Rec* misused the word *literally*, even going the extra step of exaggerating its pronunciation by saying LIT-rally (Coleman, 2013).

Reality television stars and sports stars frequently use the word *literally* instead of a more appropriate word. In 2011 when the Boston Bruins won the Stanley Cup (again), player Andrew Ference said of the victory parade, "I cannot wrap my mind around how many people were there. I literally cannot wrap my mind around it" (Boston.com, 2011). Ben Zimmer, executive producer of the Visual Thesaurus and Vocabulary.com, told the Boston.com staff, "That kind of literal mind-wrapping would be very painful indeed." Zimmer suggested other words would have better sufficed in this instance including honestly and frankly (Boston.com, 2011).

So, did Merriam-Webster change the meaning of literally? Absolutely not according to the online dictionary/thesaurus (Merriam-Webster. com, 2018a; 2018b). For example, in 1847, William Makepeace Thackeray wrote, "I *literally* blazed with wit" and Charles Dickens wrote in Nicholas Nickleby, "'Lift him out,' said Squeers, after he had *literally* feasted his eyes, in silence, upon the culprit" (Merriam-Webster.com, 2018a; 2018b).

Merriam-Webster notes the figurative use of *literally* may be annoying but it has been in use for a long time. Of course, the grammar cops began commenting soon after Merriam-Webster.com posted its article saying, "The dictionary is literally wrong," or "Our poor language, I'm figuratively about to hurl" (Merriam-Webster.com, 2018a; 2018b).

Every major dictionary includes a literal and an intensifying definition of the word *literally*. The metaphoric use of *literally* is ubiquitous and the war wages on. Because the word is misused by everyone from President Obama to Tamra Judge of the *Real Housewives of Orange County*, grammar purists worry the figurative definition will eventually eradicate the literal definition. They have good reason for concern because it has happened before. Pervasive public misuse of a word *can* change its meaning. In his essay *The Ongoing Tumult in English Usage*, Bryan A. Garner offers a hilarious, hyperbolic look at numerous misused words that he says represent a potential shift in the English language. None is more appropriate for this chapter than Garner's description of how a cartoon character caused a change in the meaning of the word *nimrod* (Garner, 2016).

For those born before 1950, the word *nimrod* may have a different meaning than it does for those born after 1950. Today, the word *nimrod* is pejorative, suggesting an idiot or dimwit. We have Bugs Bunny to thank for that. Yes, that carrot-munching, wise-cracking, trash-talking cartoon rabbit caused the post-1950s meaning of *nimrod* to eclipse the pre-1950s meaning (Garner, 2016).

Before 1950, *nimrod* meant *hunter*. Garner (2016) notes the word is derived from a biblical name in Genesis; *Nimrod* was a mighty huntsman. And so, before Bugs Bunny came along, people referred to great hunters as *nimrods*, which was a term of respect. Bugs Bunny's creators knew this and decided to use *nimrod* as a play on words. Bugs would sometimes call the inept hunter, Elmer Fudd, a *nimrod*. Fudd was no *Nimrod*, so calling him a great hunter should have been funny, just like calling a huge man *Tiny*. However, the public missed the irony and assumed *Nimrod* meant the same as dimwit. In modern language, rarely do you hear of a great huntsman being called *Nimrod* (Garner, 2016).

As nurse scientists, you likely will never need to use the word *Nimrod*. You will need to cohesively put together your dissertation or journal article and write an intelligible piece of work. You will choose each word judiciously, ensuring it means what you intend it to mean. You will construct each sentence skillfully, using only essential words to avoid verbosity. The first sentence of each paragraph should inform the rest of that paragraph's sentences. You will weave together those paragraphs, ensuring one flows naturally into the next. And you will try to avoid the following grammar and punctuation errors seen most often in dissertations and journal articles.

COMMON GRAMMATICAL ERRORS AND SOLUTIONS IN DISSERTATIONS

Now that we know why grammar is so important, we can look at some common errors. Some of these errors are so common, you will find examples and solutions on many editing websites. The following examples, however, are those I have personally seen in my 6 years of editing dissertations.

Long Sentences

One of the most pervasive issues is excessively long sentences. Not all long sentences are difficult to read. But for those that are, the key is to read it aloud. If you find yourself becoming confused as you listen to your own words, it is time to rewrite. Please remember this; you are not William Faulkner. The first story I read of Faulkner's was *Intruder in the Dust*. I was captivated, not by the story initially but by Faulkner's ability to write a single sentence for *pages* without coming up for air. In his 1936 novel, Absalom, Absalom!, Faulkner wrote a single sentence that spanned several pages; 1,287 words punctuated with commas and semicolons, gliding along before Faulkner exercised his option to end this river of words and use a period (Faulkner, 1936). In 1983, the Guinness Book of World records listed that sentence as the longest sentence in the English language. Then in 2001, Jonathan Coe wrote *The Rotters' Club* that contains one sentence of nearly 14,000 words (Coe, 2001). In the final section of Ed Park's (2008) novel *Personal Days*, you will find a single, stream-of-consciousness sentence of more than 16,000 words. The Publication Manual of the American Psychological Association (APA, 2010), the style and formatting bible for most nursing-related writing, suggests authors be prudent in their choice of words.

> Say only what needs to be said. The author who is frugal with words not only writes a more readable manuscript but also increases the chances that the manuscript will be accepted for publication (APA, 2010, p. 67).

Here is a sentence from a dissertation I recently edited.

> Situation monitoring examines the process of actively scanning and assessing situational elements to gain understanding or maintain awareness to support the functioning of the team and mutual support reviews the importance of having the ability to anticipate and support other team members' needs through accurate knowledge of their responsibilities and workload.

You may understand this sentence, especially if you re-read it. But why should you have to read a sentence more than once? Breaking this into two sentences makes it easier to read and ultimately, saves the reader from having to re-read the sentence so as to understand it. Here is that single sentence rewritten:

> Situation monitoring examines the process of actively scanning and assessing situational elements to gain understanding or maintain awareness to support the functioning of the team. Mutual support reviews the importance of having the ability to anticipate and support other team members' needs through accurate knowledge of their responsibilities and workload.

I merely added a period after team, removed the word "and," and capitalized the "M" in mutual, making it easier to read without changing the meaning.

Overly Complicated/Ambiguous Sentences

Again, not every complicated sentence is ambiguous or difficult to read but many are such as the sentence that follows:

This information would be used in creating and sustaining a "Prepared, Proactive Practice Team" in seeking the goal of achieving the "Improved Outcomes." The "Community" reflects the resources for the "Self-Management Support," reflecting the different types of caregivers, and the Department of Public Health establishing new guidelines in the newly published "All Facilities Letter," stating that hospitals, the "Health System," must identify the caregiver by name along with a telephone number in the patient's medical record "Clinical Information System" prior to discharging "Clinical Decision Support" the patient to the appropriate environment.

What would you suggest this author do to ensure clarity in this sentence? I suggested the writer rework this sentence, removing the quotation marks and italicizing any words he deemed necessary. I also suggested that reading this aloud would help him hear where the words become tangled.

The APA recognizes that sometimes, complicated sentences cannot be avoided. Here is what the APA suggests.

> When involved concepts require long sentences, the components should proceed logically. Direct, declarative sentences with simple, common words are usually best. (APA, 2010, p. 68)

Nonsensical Sentences

These happen, usually because of failure to read your work aloud. I say this often because the ear picks up what the eye does not. Consider the following sentence, and please, read it aloud.

> Another limitation of study that could have influenced the results is relating to the lack of normality could be the inherent difficulties associated with self-reporting surveys.

The author most likely would have heard the errors had he read the sentence aloud. Below is the edited version.

> Another limitation of the study that could have influenced the results is the inherent difficulties associated with self-reporting surveys.

Active Voice or Passive Voice?

You knew this was coming, didn't you? Passive versus active is another war waged among authors in the scientific community. Which should you use? The consensus is both.

In the active voice, the sentence focuses on the actor and often requires fewer words to convey the meaning. The active voice is clear, concise, and direct.

Johnson and Smith (2018) investigated the effect of simple carbohydrates on blood sugar levels.

Here, you know who is doing the action. Johnson and Smith. They are investigating.

In the passive voice, the focus is on the receiver of the action. Passive voice is often used when the actor is not known. Passive voice also usually requires more words to convey ideas and meaning, it is indirect, and can suggest hedging.

The effect simple carbohydrates have on blood sugar was investigated.

Here, you do not know who is doing the investigating. Perhaps the author did not think it important, or perhaps he or she failed to document the "who" during the research phase. Passive writing in instances like this do not sound authoritative.

While it is true the active voice is preferred over the passive voice, there are instances when the passive voice is more appropriate. The best use of passive voice is when the actors are not as important as the receivers of the action. Many scientific authors and editors agree the passive voice is most useful in the methods section because the steps taken are more important that those taking the steps. For example, it would sound better to write, "A catheter was inserted for post-operative bladder irrigation" rather than, "We inserted a catheter for post-operative bladder irrigation." Your guiding principle should be clarity. Think about the information the reader needs to know and choose the proper voice.

The APA and the American Medical Association (AMA) suggest the use of both voices as needed.

> APA prefers the active voice. "The passive voice is acceptable in expository writing and when you want to focus on the object or recipient of the action. (APA, 2010, p. 77)
>
> AMA recommends that in general, authors should use the active voice, except in instances in which the author is unknown or the interest focuses on what is acted upon. (Iverson, Christiansen, Flanagin, & JAMA and Archives Journals Staff, 2007)

Verb Tenses

The tense of the verb expresses the time at which the action described by the verb takes place. The major tenses are past, present, and future. (See Appendix 11.1 for more examples).

Here is what the APA suggests in terms of use of tenses.

> Use the past tense or the present perfect tense for the literature review and the description of the procedure if the discussion is of past events. (APA, 2010, p. 65)

The simple past tense is used when the action was completed in the past (e.g., Smith's 1998 study showed a high correlation between blood sugar levels and the consumption of processed grains, such as white rice).

Use the present perfect tense when the action or state either occurred at an indefinite time in the past (e.g., we have talked before), or if the action or state began in the past and continues to the present time (e.g., he has become impatient over the last hour).

The APA also suggests using past tense to describe results, and using present tense to discuss the implication of the results and to present the conclusions. (APA, 2010, p. 65).

The Word *Only*

Mignon Fogarty, best known as Grammar Girl (https://www.quicka nddirtytips.com/grammar-girl), calls the word *only* the most insidious misplaced modifier (Fogarty, 2013). Many authors, even the most experienced, often have trouble with the placement of *only*. The late journalist and grammarian James Kilpatrick devoted a column each year to *only* (Kilpatrick, 2007). Kilpatrick says the trick is to place *only* as close as possible to the word or phrase it modifies. He demonstrates the point with the following four sentences. Each sentence has a different meaning based on where *only* is placed (Kilpatrick, 2007).

1. **Only** John hit Peter in the nose. (John and no one else hit Peter in the nose.)
2. John hit **only** Peter in the nose. (There were a lot of people standing around insulting John, but Peter was the loudest, so John hit only Peter in the nose.)
3. John hit Peter **only** in the nose. (John could have hit Peter in the head or the knee, but he hit him in the nose.)
4. John **only** hit Peter in the nose. (John just hit the guy. He didn't pull out his machete and slash Peter's head off. He only *hit* Peter.)

Only is covered in APA Sixth Edition on page 81.

Common Punctuation Problems

Now we are having fun. Commas and hyphens and colons, oh my! There are numerous rules covering these innocent-looking, albeit important, punctuation marks. Questions arise as to the appropriate use of commas and when to use a semicolon rather than a colon. The intent here is to help you recognize when to use punctuation. The instructions here are from the sixth edition of the APA publication manual.

Commas

Many people believe inserting a comma is easy; add a comma wherever you would take a breath. This is true sometimes, but the real intent of commas is to add meaning to a sentence, not to prevent hyperventilation.

When to Use Commas

You must use the serial comma, also known as the Oxford comma, between elements (including before *and* and *or)* in a series of three or more items (APA, 2010, p. 88). For example: *In a study by Stacy, Newcomb, and Bentler (1991)*. . .

To set off a nonessential or nonrestrictive clause, that is, a clause that adds information to the sentence, but if removed would not change the meaning.

> *Button A, which is on the panel, controls the recording device.* If we removed *which is on the panel,* Button A would still control the recording device.

To separate two independent clauses <u>joined by a conjunction</u>.

> Incorrect example: *Smith and Jones (2010) found that simple carbohydrates cause blood sugar levels to rise quickly, whole grains like brown rice had little effect on blood sugar levels.* This is what is called a comma splice. A comma alone cannot separate two independent clauses. Adding a conjunction after the comma will rectify the error.

> Correct example: *Smith and Jones (2010) found that simple carbohydrates cause blood sugar levels to rise quickly, but whole grains, such as brown rice, had little effect on blood sugar levels.*

> To set off the year in exact dates.
> *April 18, 2018.*

Do not use commas:

> To separate month and year.
> *April 2018.*

Before an essential or restrictive clause, that is, a clause that limits or defines the material it modifies. Removing the clause would alter the meaning of the sentence.

> *The button that stops the recording device also controls the television.*

Between the two parts of a compound predicate. A compound predicate has two actions for the same subject, that is, the subject of the sentence is doing more than one action. The easiest way to identify a compound predicate is to look for two verbs connected by a conjunction:

> *All subjects completed the first phase of the experiment and returned the following week for Phase 2.*

> To separate parts of measurement.
> *8 years 2 months.*

Hyphens and Dashes

Hyphens and dashes (minus sign, en dash, and em dash) are covered in the sixth edition of the APA manual beginning on page 97. Each is typed differently.

A hyphen is typed using the minus sign on your keyboard. Do not add spaces before and after the hyphen.

Trial-by-trial analysis
An en dash is longer and thinner than a hyphen but shorter than an em dash. It is used between words of equal weight in a compound adjective. Do not use spaces between the words and the en dash. If your word processor does not have an en dash, use a regular hyphen. In Microsoft Word, you will find the en dash as follows: Insert > Symbol > More symbols > Special Character Tab.

Chicago–London flight
An em dash is longer than both a hyphen and an en dash and is used to set off an element added to amplify or to digress from the main clause. If your word processor does not have an em dash, use two hyphens with no spaces before or after. In Microsoft Word, you will find the em dash as follows: Insert > Symbol > More symbols > Special Character Tab.

Studies—published and unpublished—are included.
The most common use of the en dash and the em dash in scholarly writing is to mark parenthetical clauses and indicate a more pronounced break in the sentence than using a comma. However, both the en dash and the em dash are less formal than colons and often suggest an aside or an afterthought. The APA does not encourage excessive use of these punctuation marks.

Do not use hyphens and dashes as follows:
With a compound including an adverb ending in -ly
Widely used text
With a compound including a comparative or superlative
Higher scoring student
With common fractions used as nouns
One third of the participants

Colons

Colons call attention to themselves, so when an author uses a colon, it sends a signal to the reader to pay close attention. Colons are covered in the sixth edition of the APA manual on page 90. In the following example, the colon is used after an introductory clause that can stand on its own.

They have agreed on the outcome: Informed participants perform better than do uninformed participants.

Colons are used in ratios and proportions.

The proportion (saltwater) was 1:8.

Colons are used in references between cities of publication and publisher.

Thousand Oaks, CA: Sage

Colons are used to introduce a list, but the part of the sentence that comes before the colon must be a complete sentence.

The wine bottles were lined up on the counter in the following order: Cabernet, Chardonnay, Rosé, and Chianti.

Colons are not used after prepositions.

She had all the skills of a great nurse leader, such as dedication to her role, a great team player, and the ability to be flexible and adaptable.
The instructions for the task are to read Chapter 2. (Note there is no colon placed after "are.")

Capitalize the first word after a colon only if the sentence that follows is a complete sentence.

The author made one main point: No explanation that has been suggested so far answers all questions.

Semi-colons

Semi-colons are used to join independent clauses that are not joined by a conjunction.

The participants in the first study were paid; those in the second study were unpaid.

Semi-colons separate elements in a series that already contain commas.

The color order was red, yellow, blue; blue, yellow, red; or yellow, red, blue.
Age, M = 34.5 years, 95% Cl [29.4, 39.6]; years of education, M =10.4 [8.7, 12.1]; and weekly income, M =612 [622, 702].

A Word on Spell Checkers and Citation Managers

Software-based spell checkers and citation managers are helpful tools, but they are not infallible. It is a good idea to use them but not rely on them. Citation managers are only as good as the individual entering the data. Even after the citation manager formats your in-text citations and list of references, I recommend that you still review each entry in your document for proper formatting. I often find numerous errors, particularly in the list of references. In fact, this is usually the section where I spend the most time editing and ensuring what is in the in-text citations appears in the list of references and vice versa.

THE DREADED "E" WORD—EDITING

You are finally finished. You have set aside your masterpiece for a period of time (this will depend on the amount of time between finishing the document and your deadline). The longer you can leave it, the easier it will be to find errors when you do finally return to it because you will return to it with fresh eyes.

When you are ready, read through the document slowly and preferably aloud. Look and listen for style, consistency, and cohesion. Once the document flows the way you want, make one more pass and concentrate on the grammar and punctuation. The reason I suggest you wait until the end to make grammar and punctuation edits is because during your first pass, you will likely make major revisions in your work; sometimes you will remove or rewrite entire paragraphs. It would be a waste of your time to have edited for grammar and punctuation when, in the end, you removed or changed large sections of your work. Authors sometimes read their work sentence-by-sentence beginning at the end of the document. While this does not help with cohesion, it will help you find more spelling, grammar, and punctuation errors.

Some of you prefer to do your own editing and I applaud you for that. As an editor, I catch almost all errors on my first pass when I am reading the work of others. But when I edit my own writing, I do not see as many mistakes. That is why I encourage you to have someone else review your work, whether you hire an editor to do it or promise your buddy a nice dinner if he or she reviews it. Your work will be better for it. The other person has never seen the work so he or she is more likely to catch spelling, punctuation, formatting, and grammar errors. Your designee is also not attached to the work, so it is much easier to cut out unnecessary words, including those words that comprise what you think is the most beautiful, creatively constructed sentence you have ever written. To paraphrase Johnny Cochrane, if it does not fit, you must dump it.

CONCLUSION

This chapter introduced the importance of grammar and the necessity to use it correctly. Some companies now require job applicants to take grammar tests. If you worry about taking those tests, you will find many grammar-related websites that offer free tests. One of the best is Grammar Monster. Grammar Monster has a website (https://www

.grammar-monster.com/), a You Tube channel (https://www.youtube
.com/channel/UChHAB-I_VMnYtXFRnXr_VLA/featured), and is active on Twitter (https://twitter.com/grammarmonster?ref_src=tws
rc%5Egoogle%7Ctwcamp%5Eserp%7Ctwgr%5Eauthor), and Facebook
(https://www.facebook.com/GrammarMonster/).

We also discussed misused words and how some of those words become officially recognized in the dictionary after frequent misuse in everyday speech. The meaning of the word *nimrod* changed because television
viewers misunderstood a Bugs Bunny joke. Traditionally, the word *enormity* means horrific as in *the enormities of war,* but today, the word is used
more to describe immenseness, as in *the enormity of the job.* We discussed
the most common grammar-related errors seen in nursing PhD dissertations and suggestions for correction. Finally, and most importantly, we
talked about how poor grammar can negatively impact your credibility.

If editing your work makes you feel like you just stepped on something the producers of Fear Factor devised, relax. Editors were created
just for you. Your work, and the work of all authors, will benefit from
having someone else review it. It is likely what you prefer, anyway. You
are a researcher, born to find better ways for humankind to progress.
Congratulations. You are *literally* a *Nimrod*!

FURTHER READINGS

Callihan, E. L. (1957). *Grammar for journalists.* Philadelphia, PA: Chilton
Book.

Fogerty, M. (2008). *Grammar Girl's quick and dirty tips for better writing.*
New York, NY: St. Martin's Griffin. (Also, Mignon has a blog and
podcast at https://www.quickanddirtytips.com/grammar-girl.)

Fogerty, M. (2011). *Grammar Girl presents the ultimate writing guide for
students.* Logan, IA: Perfection Learning Corporation. (This is a great
guide once you get past the cheesy section titles, which include
Subject-Verb Agreement: Cannot We All Just Get Along; Reflexive
Pronouns: Dancing with *Myself;* and my Favorite, Comma, Comma,
Comma, Comma, Comma, Chameleon.)

Garner, B. A. (2016). *The Chicago guide to grammar, usage, and punctuation.*
Chicago, IL: University of Chicago Press.

Lester, M., & Beason, L. (2012). *The McGraw-Hill handbook of English grammar and usage,* (2nd Ed.). New York, NY: McGraw-Hill Education.

Norris, M. (2015). *Between you and me: Confessions of a comma queen.* New
York, NY: W. W. Norton & Company.

Straus, J., Kaufman, L., & Stern, T. (2014). *The blue book of grammar and
punctuation: An easy–to–use guide with clear rules, real–world examples,
and reproducible quizzes,* (11th Ed.). San Francisco, CA: Jossey-Bass.

Truss, L. (2009). *Eats, shoots & leaves.* London, UK: Profile Books.

Walsh, B. (2004). *The elephants of style: A trunkload of tips on the big issues and gray areas of contemporary American English.* New York, NY: McGraw-Hill Education.

REFERENCES

American Psychological Association. (2010). *The publication manual of the American Psychological Association.* (6th ed.). Washington, DC: The American Psychological Association.

Boston.com. (2011, July). Literally the most misused word. Retrieved from https://www.boston.com/culture/lifestyle/2011 /07/19/literally -the-most-misused-word

Coe, J. (2001). *The Rotters' Club.* New York, NY: Vintage Books.

Coleman, D. (2013, August). According to the dictionary, "literally" now also means "figuratively." Salon.com. Retrieved from https://www .salon.com/2013/08/22/according_to_the_dictionary_literally _now_also_means_figuratively_newscred

Faulkner, W. (1936). *Absalom, Absalom!* New York, NY: Random House.

Fogarty, M. (2013). "Only": The most insidious misplaced modifier. Retrieved from https://www.quickanddirtytips.com/education/ grammar/%E2%80%9Conly%E2%80%9D-the-most-insidious-mis placed-modifier

Garner, B. A. (2016). The ongoing tumult in English usage. In *Garner's Modern American English Usage* (4th ed.). New York, NY: Oxford University Press.

Iverson, C., Christiansen, S., Flanagin, A., & JAMA and Archives Journals Staff (Eds.). (2007). *AMA manual of style: A guide for authors and editors* (10th ed.). New York, NY: Oxford University Press.

Kilpatrick, J. (2007, January). *If we could only get this one right.* The Eugene Register-Guard. Retrieved from https://news.google.com/ newspapers?id=4WBWAAAAIBAJ&sjid=tfADAAAAIBAJ& pg=6697,2895111&hl=en

Merriam-Webster.com. (2018a). *Literally.* Retrieved from https://www .merriam-webster.com/dictionary/literally?utm_campaign=sd& utm_medium=serp&utm_source=jsonld

Merriam-Webster.com. (2018b). *Did we change the definition of 'literally'?* Retrieved from https://www.merriam-webster.com/words-at-play/ misuse-of-literally

Park, E. (2008). *Personal days.* New York, NY: Random House

Wiens, K. (2012, July). I will not hire people who use poor grammar. Here's why. *Harvard Business Review.* Retrieved from https://hbr .org/2012/07/i-wont-hire-people-who-use-poo

APPENDIX 11.1 SIMPLE AND PERFECT VERB TENSES

Verb Forms	Tense	How Used	How Created	Example
Simple tenses Action that takes place at a single point or moment in time.	**Past**	Action completed at a past moment in time. The primary vehicle for all narration that deals with time events	Base + "-d" or "-ed"	I walked.
	Present (base form)	Action occurring now, at the present moment in time (but we use progressive present tense for that) Something done regularly Statements of fact or generalizations (scientific fact or generalized truth) Discuss literature, film, art, and music. Introduce a quotation, summary, paraphrase Indicate future time	Third person singular (he, she) = Base + "s" All others = Base	I walk/he walks (for charity). Progressive present tense = I am walking.
	Future	A future moment in time	"Will" + Base Present progressive + future time signal Or modal verbs: "can, may, must, shall" "could, might, should, would"	I will/would walk. I can/could walk. I'm walking on Friday. I may/might walk. I must walk. I shall/should walk.
	Past participle	Used in perfect tenses, passive voice, and past participial phrases (used as adjectives)	Base + "-ed"	An endangered species.
	Infinitive ("to" base)	The form of the verb preceded by "to"	"To" + Base	To walk
	Present participle	Used to form progressive tenses	Base + "-ing"	Walking

(continued)

Verb Forms	Tense	How Used	How Created	Example
Perfect Tenses Actions that span a period of time. Action completed before a particular time, action, or event. Action begun in the past and continues to the present. Uses verb "**Have**" in some form, + **Past Participle**.	**Past Perfect**	An action that began at a more distant point in the past and ended at a more recent point in the past. Used to indicate which of two past actions occurred first.	"Had" + Past Participle	I had walked to the store. The plane had left before I arrived.
	Present Perfect	An action that began in the past and continues up to the present time. Continuously is key word. Also used for completed action with indefinite time.	"Have/has" + Past participle	I have walked to the store. I have been to Rome.
	Future Perfect	An action that begins in the future and ends by some more distant point in the future. Emphasizes "no later than" time of completion of the future action.	"Will have" + Past participle	I will have walked to the store.

INDEX

Printed in the United States
By Bookmasters